TREAT YOURSELF

A STEP-BY-STEP APPROACH TO SUPERCHARGE
YOUR IMMUNE SYSTEM AND CREATE BETTER
HEALTH AND WELLNESS FOR YOUR FAMILY

Dr. Alan Trites

Copyright©2020 by Dr. Alan Trites

ISBN: 978-1-7350685-0-3

Dedication

It is with great pride that I dedicate this manual to my wife Angela, our lovely children, my parents who allowed me to beat my own path, and the giants who put me on their shoulders and made this knowledge available to me; Milt, Gordon and David.

Table of Contents

INTRODUCTION

I f there was a simple practice you could do to help yourself when you were hurt or sick that could make you better, wouldn't you want to learn it?

Of course, these are conditions not bad enough to warrant a trip to the emergency room. But I want you to help yourself before you need that trip. It is my vision not to let anyone I know or will know become a statistic by not being responsible and taking action for their health. This is only a gateway into igniting a fire in your desire to learn, take action and spread this knowledge. The body is in fact the great healer, and we are only the mediators to aid in its speedy recovery.

It is my wish to provide insight to these possibilities, to provide you with ideas for you and your family's care with easy things to do at home, but not be a replacement for sound medical care. Also, it is to provide education on laboratory tests that would help you with communicating with your doctor. This book is my way of providing a simple educational tool for each of us to gain a role and be the authority in our health.

Why you?

Have you ever had a headache and put your hands on your head? Or put your hands on your back to provide relief and support? Have you ever hurt a body part and placed your hand on that body part while it was in pain?

Why did you do that? Is this motion of touching oneself proven and published as valid? Can you imagine a pharmaceutical commercial with the message that it is better to touch an area that hurts instead of reaching for a medication?

Most of us have placed our hands on ourselves to make something that hurt feel better. Was it because your mother taught you to do so? The answer is most likely no. These "receptors" where you touch are very important concepts when treating yourself. What you were doing is connecting a circuit for your brain to understand what's going on. Your brain works fast, roughly 500,000 times faster than your iPad [1]

You make more complex calculations for what is required for life than the fastest computer. Although the internet and supercomputers now have more storage. These include your movement, digestion, thoughts, and physiology. All are a series of calculations by your brain. When you touch yourself for pain, thought, or pleasure, you are sending multiple signals to your brain. If it hurts, your brain receives the message on where it hurts and also feels what is going on. Should something be cold or hot, each one of those signals goes to a different part of the brain. If you actually feel better, that is yet another part of the brain.

And you also need to remember if you did something clumsy and to not do it again. Your clumsy signals go to yet another part. There's a lot of mechanical and chemical messages from your brain to your body when you move. This includes where to send blood and where to cut blood off with movement. The importance is if the joint moving is getting enough blood and the stagnant joint is not. Blood supply management and spatial awareness is how to keep your balance. Then, when you want exercise, your brain communicates with receptors enhancing your ability to perform.[2]

The majority of sensation and pain go through specific receptors in the body known as mechanoreceptors. These receptors are like the important sensors in your car. They input to your brain. Let's take your car for example. One sensor might alert you that a door is open, another might inform you that you are about to hit something. Assuming your body has hit something, the majority of the information received by the brain will be acknowledged and ignored. Only the biggest and most important signals get utilized.[3]

3

A proper functioning brain deals with the importance of each signal. A malfunctioning brain reacts to everything. This is called anxiety, ADD, or ADHD. It could also be low latent autism. This is where there are too many signals firing in the brain leading to emotional overwhelm, overload, and shutdown. We have all been there before under the right circumstances. I will teach you a great deal about the input of your signals to treat yourself. You harness the power to heal yourself and help your family. You have a hidden potential that most likely has not been explained to you in this way. It is my goal to provide you tools so that you can wield this knowledge and improve your health.[4]

How did this come to me, and why should you read further?

Decades ago, I got into alternative medicine more as a curiosity to explain how it could work. I was finishing my clinical laboratory science degree and had access to several medical doctors to ask questions to. I chose to ask these doctors because I had sat in on procedures and had a good rapport. I first asked the orthopedic doctors what they thought of chiropractors. The orthopedic doctor only thought chiropractors stretched a joint but couldn't explain how. Then I asked the pain management clinic about acupuncture. The pain clinic doctors said that some people feel better, but there's no science to prove it. Then I asked the endocrinologist and allergist about homeopathy. I was hoping for a better response because they were using hormones and allergy shots and compounds. These therapies were the closest to homeopathy that I could find. Both the endocrinologist and allergist said their process was different but couldn't tell me how or why.

The doctors I interviewed about alternative medicine were not dismissive, nor did they have a negative attitude toward them. What I learned during my inquiry—and I mean this with respect—was that they had no idea about any of these alternative professions. No offense to them.

My experience with professionals is that most stay in their lane and don't seek eclectic knowledge. After my info quest, I started some deep research of my own. There are actually thousands of peer-reviewed published research papers on alternative medicine listed on PubMed. This is a medical publication website run by the United States National Library of Medicine. It has strict rules and regulations about how and what gets published. These rules include peer-reviewed papers, settings, sample size, types of studies, and outcomes. In other words, you can't submit a paper or literature review without a great deal of effort.

My journey into alternative medicine began with learning basic acupuncture. When I was running competitively, either between races or sometimes during, I used acupressure points to get me through my efforts. I used the points for pain, sore muscles, and recovery. The points I used I had learned from Chinese and Japanese acupuncture.

Then I added further studies in auriculotherapy, Korean hand acupuncture and Meridian graphing. This became a hobby because my real job was working in a medical laboratory. During an incredibly busy weekend at the E.R., we had dozens of heart attack admissions around midnight. I discovered with my acupuncture studies that the 11 P.M-1 A.M. timeframe is exactly what the Chinese had written about 6,000 years ago for the heart! Some of my co-workers were quick to dismiss that fact due to people waiting to go into the E.R.[5]

Those are logical Western medicine opinions, but are not 100% true. That said in our hospital we were not allowed to go to lunch between 11 P.M. and 1 A.M yet that was the only time not permitted for the entire day. Coincidence? It was when most heart attack admissions occurred there. Is it possible the ancients observed these time phenomenons? It's it possible there are complementary options to our current medical health care? Can these old techniques work and can you be precise in your assessment like I was in the lab? For me, things started making sense in the laboratory when the acupuncture charts lined up with current physiology.

The heart has its lowest energy at 11 P.M.-1 AM according to the Chinese acupuncture cycle. It is thought because we are at rest and low activity, or at least supposed to be resting. Well, that makes sense for a heart attack. If it has the least amount of blood supply during 11 P.M- 1 A.M. according to the Chinese energy cycle. Then that would be the time most susceptible to lack of oxygen leading to a heart attack. Over the years there were many other similarities. But I couldn't stop there. I had to understand how acupuncture could tie into blood tests. Can you treat an acupuncture point to change a blood test result? I was quite shocked to see that you can. Not only can you change a blood test marker, you can also change something called heart rate variability, or HRV.[6]

Blood tests and HRV are very hard if not impossible to cheat. I have benefitted in my education learning functional medicine, functional nutrition, functional neurology, genetics, methyl genetics, and epigenetic expression to name a few. I discovered there were three variables that came along with pathology. These exist regardless of condition or disease. You have to address inflammation, swelling, and blood sugar. It didn't matter the type of doctor or technique.

Most doctors were addressing at best one variable. When I figured out I could address all three variables, I learned something profound. I learned to do a great job at preventing disease and minimizing it in those who already have it.

Medicine—or more specifically emergency care medicine—is wonderful and lifesaving, but where's the prevention? Yes, accidents do happen. But the majority of cardiovascular disease, obesity, diabetes, and many chronic illnesses are preventable. Our nation due to our lack of education for health, how to maintain health, and what starves us of our health makes us number 1 in spending and 37th in world health.[7] [8]

In general, Americans go to the doctor after a problem has occurred. Isn't this too late? Wouldn't you want to enhance health outcomes and promote prevention? In a perfect world, the combination of medicine and natural medicine would be an ideal solution. I'm a realist. There are conditions that are so far degenerated, or idiopathic—meaning no one knows why or how it occurs—that medical intervention is the only reasonable course of action.

Hippocrates once said "let your food be your medicine and your medicine be your food." We will dive deep into this in future chapters. Your health is interconnected to many other processes in life. To erect a home, one must have good building materials and a solid foundation. If you have a good foundation but lousy materials, then the home won't be that sturdy. Or if you have great materials on quicksand, you're also out of luck. I say you need both.

I will also talk about specific food programs for your genes and specific conditions. Also, I will provide a general overview of the current marketed diet programs and how they may or may not apply to you. I can roughly estimate that I have spent around 10,000 hours in education and invested well over $1,000,000. It is not only in one genre or one type of therapy. I do my best to keep looking and understand new and old approaches. This is because more than one way for someone to help themselves exists. Or, you may respond wonderfully to one therapy and tank on something that is sufficient for the masses.

I observed in my education that there are three fundamental pillars to heal yourself. You need to address each.

A guru or two might say mind, body, spirit. Okay. That makes sense until you get hit by a truck.

It's difficult to enlighten yourself when you are injured so badly that you depend on others to use the restroom. But importance is all relevant. If you were a neurologist, you would make your brain the most important. I'm not advocating that your brain does not need to function. You need to have a complementary attitude. In order for your brain to function effective it must have proper nutrition and quality stimulation. As you can see, it's more than staring at the brain.

Most people are addressing one or more of these pillars whether that is on their own or with their doctor. One approach is to take medicine. Another to see a nutritionist or dietician for what to eat. Perhaps you take supplements or a combination with nutrition and medication. This approach is medication-food-supplements otherwise known as nutrients. Okay, that makes sense. But how do you expect my oral aid to go through my mouth and fix my broken toe or my headaches? Is my supplement psychic or clairvoyant?

A second approach might be to see a physical therapist, chiropractor, acupuncturist, or a bodywork person. Well now, that doctor is generally working on the area that hurts. But think about this. Explain to me how their treatment is to remain fixed if you don't have the building blocks of nutrients to heal?

The third approach is to work on your education and yourself through brain work. You stimulate your brain through eye exercises, reading, learning a new skill or new language, balance exercises, or mental games. How many people are doing all three? The answer is not many.

There was a time I observed or helped out other doctors from varying disciplines. I would often see that after a patient got a treatment, they would leave the office and get fast food. When I saw this, I would tell the treating doctor to fire their patient.

They would ask, "Why?"

I'd explain, "Because you did all that good work, and within ten minutes, they are ruining their treatment. You can't be responsible for that!"

What happens when someone goes to the dentist, and on the way home, they get a soft drink to get that taste out of their mouth? They're ruining their treatment! This happens all the time, regardless of doctor. Sometimes a patient is too quick to go back to exercise or other activities before their joints are healed. Or, the doctor didn't take the time to explain how long it takes tissue to heal.

We are going to work on three pillars of health with none being more important than the other. All three pillars of health working together make your brain work more effectively. If you can't move, your brain slows down. If you can't think, your brain slows down. If you can't digest or you eat the wrong food, your brain slows down. In short, your brain slows down for each pillar. If your brain works slow you don't enjoy life, taste food, have drive and function. Chapters 5 and parts of 4 and 6 and consists of pillar one: focus on your brain and immune system.

The second pillar is chemistry with the majority consisting of nutrition. Without proper nutrition, your structure cannot repair and grow. Without nutrition, your thought process and brain function will limit capability. Chapters 7-10 focus here. Again, it's not more important than the other pillars, but it has the most variables.

The third pillar defined is structural health which consists of mechanoreceptors, exercise, flexibility, strength, and coordination. The third pillar is also your psyche which contains brain function not in the first pillar. This includes a part of your brain that runs the autonomic nervous system (ANS). The ANS consists of two parts known as parasympathetic and sympathetic. Your spirit can be your religious conviction and/or mental and emotional connections. Your thoughts that can inhibit or enhance your physiology. As a heads up, structure denotes function and is very easy to follow. Chapters 11-13 focus on this.[9]

You are the best person to be your primary care provider. You are the most qualified with life experiences on the beautiful being that is you. You are the one who's responsible to assess your life and to live a life of wellness.

Please forgive me if I sound like the guru or someone that preaches "it's only positivity in thought" with the hopes of creating something that you do not possess. Here's what I can tell you back in the world of reality: When people give up on themselves, things tend to spiral down.

When people ignore their health, so many other facets of their life suffer.

You can have physical pain or joint pain that decreases your movement, or your ability to do things with your family or friends. You might have a mental or emotional pain that changes your social output, interactions, energy levels, and drive. And you can have chemical pain that makes it difficult to go out to eat, choose a perfume, or make food for people.

I don't like the cliché that pain is weakness leaving your body when I can appreciate pain as a warning sign.

13

Once you understand it yourself, then you can make the changes in the energetic systems of your body. You can address the three pillars of health.

Many of the topics in this book are from the most common symptoms and conditions observed. I took my experience through two decades of hospital employment and private practice. In 2007, I spread my practices throughout the country and it became impossible to see patients immediately when they desired. When they had recurring symptoms and I couldn't see them for a month, what could they do?

The true definition of doctor is teacher.

It was then I began telemedicine, in 2005. To help the lives of many patients in search of relief, I needed a go between until they could seek care. I had to teach them what to treat because I may not see them for 6-8 weeks with both of our schedules. It was then my purpose was to create a self-help manual and an explanatory book to simplify treatment so patients could treat themselves until they saw me or their doctor. This became my mantra.

In the beginning, the self-help manual was awfully basic. It was more metaphysical than physical. The basic premise was understanding that nothing is certain in physiology. At least, not as we perceive it to be from a medical point of view. The body is in fact the great healer and we are only the mediators to aid in its speedy recovery.

Please ask questions and read all the literature you can find. I insist you read about each product from both the manufacturer and research if it exists. I will be making updates in the future as new and interesting topics arise through my webinars and live classes. Please join our healthy habits alerts to keep ahead on new topics.

Enjoy and Be well,

Dr. Alan Trites

"We make a living by what we get, but we make a life by what we give." Winston Churchill

CHAPTER 1

Is It Possible a New Approach Is Needed?

S ince I began to take an active role in health care for myself and others 30 years ago, a lot has changed. It's been 20 years since I first licensed in health care. Some things have changed. Yearly, there are more pharmaceuticals, more advertisements, more disease labels, (oppositional defiant disorder comes to mind), requiring long-term and/or life-long medication. We live in a country that has one of the best profit based, high-tech, crisis-care medicine. Yet, it has become costly and at times dangerous. Many can't afford mediocre health insurance. Those fortunate to have insurance have increasing premiums, higher co-pays and more denials, or you are not allowed to pick your doctor. Our system requires them to pay for it out of pocket even when they're supposed to have coverage. If you want to be on top of your health, you need to invest in yourself. Obsolete is the sit back and wait approach, praying you have insurance coverage.[10] [11]

There are more individuals looking for alternative approaches and solutions than when I first began by far. But, there is still as the majority thought in our society with the 'take a pill for what you ill' mentality. Many of the topics in this book are from the most common symptoms and conditions observed. Your body is a great healer and we can aid in its recovery with what you are going to learn. I want to provide insight to these possibilities, to provide you with ideas for you and your family's care with easy things to do at home,

I want you to know that health is not an absence of symptoms. It is a combination of millions of energies packets that somehow create life. I will provide the basics. Learning this information could take several lifetimes, at least for me. Who knows, this may still only be the beginning of our knowledge.

This book is a holistic approach to personal health. It is for those who may or may not have any previous knowledge on how their body works. You are an exceptional person. You have unique biochemistry. You have an individual bioelectric energy signature that makes each of us special. If you don't believe even part of this, then don't buy the latest iPhone with the thumb print or face recognition. They open for you on bioelectric energy signatures.

Disease is not limited to a lock and key or mechanistic process as Newtonian physics and current medicine researches and publishes. In general, physicists and medicine have been unable to explain holistic medicine. Medicine utilizes Newtonian physics where alternative does not. Alternative medicine is more quantum physics without being full-blown quantum physics. Just speaking that seems complicated enough! Newtonian physics explains the mechanistic effects of our world. These are basic physiology, medication, gravity, and propulsion to name a few.

But then it gets entirely complicated and leaves science scratching its head. Important characteristics such as nerve conduction, thoughts, prayer, and love that violate the laws of Newtonian physics. It is because these actions are more in the realm of quantum physics and are more influential to your existence. Medicine cannot explain love, thought, and prayer, and you cannot patent them. But they exist.

Alternative practitioners are quick to omit man-made ideas, but they exist. I can't imagine where I would be without blood tests to confirm an exam, or a picture to show a broken leg. What I'm saying is you need them both, and at certain times in your life you will need one more than another.

What are we?

Everything we do, eat, sleep, move, and think is a process of electromagnetic change. Again, your brain can do more complex calculations than any supercomputer known to man. And it can do it in milliseconds. This function, called quantum changes or the quantum way, is essential for life to be possible as we currently experience. Quantum energy are very small packets of energy. You may recall some of the names.

Sometimes I start by asking a group, What are we? People shout, "Bones," "Ligaments," "Organs," or "Brain cells."

Yes, cells. What are cells made of?

Going back to middle school, we learned about organelles such as the mitochondria, Golgi apparatus, cytosol, and nucleus. Yes, what is in the nucleus? DNA.

Perfect. Let's graduate to high school. What is DNA made from? Code bases from adenine (A), guanine (G), cytosine (C), and thymine (T). And those are what? Molecules. Which are made from what? Atoms that have their mass stored in the nucleus. Which consist of what? Protons, electrons, and neutrons. These are subatomic particles and do not contain mass. Subatomic particles function by even smaller energy packets known as quarks. If we choose, we can go on for a bit more, getting smaller and smaller and smaller.

But, let's talk physics for a brief minute and then we can put it to rest for the remainder of this book. Newtonian physics is based on mass, period. You don't have to remember middle and high school science. From the above, we can agree that for the most part you've heard of it, right? So what percentage is the mass part of the atom? It's not 50% as most diagrams show, 10%, or even 1%. The actual mass portion of an atom, something we can all agree we are composed of, is .01%. The other 99.9% are the subatomic particles. My point is that we are a huge percentage of subatomic particles not containing mass. Modern science using Newtonian physics focuses on mass only. Perhaps those other concepts that help move energy around may actually be beneficial to a human consisting of 99.9% energy. Subtle energies of the body are your basic entrance to quantum physics and the purpose of this self-help manual.

This understanding of you is why you are the best person to be your primary care provider. You are the most qualified with life experiences on the beautiful being that is you. You are the one who's responsible to assess your life and to live a life of wellness. You get to have a say in what is happening. Once you understand yourself then you can make the changes in the energetic systems of your body. You also will have better knowledge in how to communicate with your doctor when you need one. You can change your physiology with thought, diet, movement, and self-treatment.

Regarding thought, there is benefit in a positive attitude and expecting great outcomes. We wouldn't have sports or other professions if no one expected a negative outcome, and we certainly wouldn't consider having children if there was no positive benefit to our outcome.

Marketing and advertising companies are well-versed in this pillar by manipulating your thoughts. They can change your opinion of food, make-up, self-care, cars, and medications by showing happy, care-free people having a great time while having unlimited income free of debilitating diseases.

Indulge me for a minute as I take you through a story to explain this. Pretend that you are in the desert and it's very, very hot. You haven't had a thing to drink. Your lips are dry and peeling, your mouth is dying for thirst and your tongue is stuck to your mouth. Take a moment to embrace your thirst and imagine what that would feel like. Put yourself in the desert and feel how miserable you are.

Now I come along and I can see that you're parched. The only item I have with me is one lemon. I slice it in half and I know that I can't give it all to you because you'll become sick. So, I ask you to close your eyes and lean your head back. As you struggle to peel your lips apart and stick out your dry tongue, I squeeze the lemon, and two drops land on the tip of your tongue. I'm going to stop here. This isn't about a desert or lemons. Make an observation. For the majority of people reading, they have created saliva. You created a physiological response. Saliva is the very first part of your digestive system. Within seconds your digestion is firing and yet it's all from thought.

So, it's true. Thought can create physiology, and you need to understand food manufacturers are very aware of this. When it comes to your health, thought changes physiology. The same can be provided for getting you to purchase a car or medication.

The Reality

The pharmaceutical industry spends billions in drug advertising, and billions more educating doctors on their uses and side effects. There are concerns that it is not "FDA approved," or there is not enough medical research to substantiate a claim or benefit to a treatment. Yet, once a death occurs in natural medicine, the FDA appears to get involved. Furthermore, the FDA doesn't deem it necessary to test any claims against natural medicinal aids unless of course it creates a large problem, like death.

Is that fair? Do they have bigger issues with regulating medications that have a toxic level resulting in many deaths? Consider malpractice insurance. A chiropractor compared with an OBGYN. One pays $1200 a year and the other averages over $100,000 a year.[12] Why the gross discrepancy? One profession gets sued 86% of the time, even if it's 1 out of 1000 clients. While considered scary to some, the rate of breaking necks or causing strokes is 1 out of 5,000,000 clients. By the way, that stroke is three times more likely to happen when getting your hair washed at the hair salon! Yes, the salon has insurance as well.

Why doesn't the FDA take more of a stance on natural medicine? The main reasons for this is the FDA is underfunded and understaffed. It cannot take the time to test these with the large number of pharmaceuticals implemented and tested through various trials. The vast number of natural supplements don't cause the harm or potential loss of life that can occur with pharmaceuticals. Moreover, a large number of doctors, medical and even so-called natural health physicians, have a hard time understanding that often simple and safe alternatives exist. These intelligent doctors needed to spend years learning how to administer a non-lethal dose of dangerous medications. You want them to know this information.

Then, there is a greater understanding of what actually occurs in the body. "In vitro" means in a test tube. So, here's some truth that creates disapproving smirks directed toward me. Most medical literature including the "scientific method" that you learned in school has parts taken out of the body and studied. In contrast, the "in vivo" test means in the body.

How many "in vivo" tests are evaluated on humans for reactions of medications? The answer is less than one percent.

What is the average number of medications an American is on? Seven.[13]

So, how many of these patient's dosage, chemistry, lifespan, side effects are only a best guess but not actual science? How do you know that your medication doesn't affect another system? How do you know you're gaining benefits versus a side effect and how do we know one medication isn't influencing another?

I'll let you take it from here. In vitro test takes a part out of the body and explains that this is truth. This is the same as IV fertilization.

Parts of cells are taken out and placed back in. However, the body is a group of systems communicating neurologically, chemically, and more importantly the true basis for life—bioelectrically.

Let's start with the topic of medications known as non-steroidal anti-inflammatory drugs or NSAIDs. There're some people who respond to salicylic acid (Aspirin) and have no response to acetaminophen (Tylenol), or ibuprofen (Advil) and vice versa. Why? It is because we have unique biochemistry. We have a different set of genes and we can take similar yet different substances with different results. We could have friends that we work out with and do the same workout. We could eat the same foods without our spouse and children. Yet, we respond and recover differently.

Most doctors including alternative natural doctors have only one tool and their toolbox. So, if the only tool your doctor has is a hammer, everything to them looks like a nail.

This is why I study for about 30 hours a week. The information at times is overwhelming. Because there are new emerging ideas, new tools and new research, I often need to update the way I practice. This is because not everybody responds to the same medication.

Not everybody responds to chiropractic, massage, or acupuncture, nor nutrition, or physical therapy, alone or combined.

Some patients need brain-balancing exercises or memory games. Others need electrical stimulation, gentle exercise, or high intensity training. **Some patients need it all.**

So, you need to have many tools in your toolbox. You will learn tools as you continue to read and then be able to apply those tools in this self-help manual.

It is a fact that simpler, preventable methods are not passed through generations or deemed "non-scientific." Unfortunately, the scientific basis for United States health is close to the number one cause of death.

According to Death by Medicine (2004), nine million Americans were unnecessarily hospitalized, and tens of millions were inappropriately prescribed antibiotics. Two point two million have adverse drug reactions to properly prescribed medications, and 783,936 deaths were caused by conventional medicine.[14]

That number was from sixteen years ago, it continues to rise, and yet our country was not shut down. We need to be aware enough to make a change for health.

Currently, the fastest growing disabled group is not the baby boomer generation, but instead those prescribed antidepressants, anti-anxiety, and other psychotropic medications, from Anatomy of an Epidemic.[15] This isn't a group with massive dosing or the wrong medication. They consist of the correct dose and medication!

Hippocrates, the Father of Medicine, said, "Let your food be your medicine and let your medicine be your food."

Health begins from your own grown farm if you can, not a pharmacy. Do you grow your own food, eat organic, or read labels? Do you eat out often or purchase packaged foods? If it's at the store, does it really qualify as edible?

There are many studies that show how our diet influences our health and our genetic expression. It is not everything, as we must have brainpower and exercise. It is not an exact science. If you choose to educate and do it yourself, it is my expectation and experience your health will improve. You can start to change even if you do a little. Every action is a step in the right direction.

The bias against natural medicine is there, and not enough is published in mainstream medical journals. No kidding. That's because it's not contemporary or congruent with medical influence.[16]Natural medicine can prevent and treat illness and promote optimal health. It is not a complete mystery. Because of the multi-factor influences on each human, it's not an exact science either.

Again, the current science we are all taught in school is not based from quantum physics, but instead Newtonian physics. Natural medicine has no true universal accepted position or definition. What is it then? It is the use of diet or dietary modifications. It's nutritional supplements, natural hormones, herbs, and other natural substances. It's exercise, thought, and physical treatments. There is no question medicine is great at emergency care, but the medical mainstream as a whole has been overlooking something important, especially in chronic conditions.

Patients continue to come into offices with a myriad of symptoms. They can express physical and mental problems. Many of my patients have failed to respond to the best and current medications and therapies offered. That's frustrating. My alternative colleagues and I often hear from patients, "I've been to so many doctors and I still don't feel better." Or "I've spent $30,000 and you're the first one who's given me an answer and has helped me feel better."

Why? I took a chance to learn and understand there are other ways to enhance the health of my patient other than evaluating only the presence or absence of disease. I've been in their shoes going from doctor to doctor in search of answers. Not one technique, medication, surgery, therapy or nutrient will help all people, Let's bring this into our new reality.

Consider the latest coronavirus where, if you have antibodies or are infused with antibodies, you have a chance for recovery. The antibodies lock onto the virus in the immune system by way of natural killer T-cells that come along and kill it. It is unfortunate that not everyone has the perfect response.[17] [18]

Here are the missing elements regarding how a person responds or not. Factors including how a person eats, sleeps, exercises, and handles stress are vitally important. Can they make an immune response if infused were the antibodies for Covid-19 or a different coronavirus? Will it have the same effect? Have they taken care of themselves, whether that's the previous week, month, or year? Do they have any environmental factors influencing their health? Do they smoke, consume too much alcohol, or have they had a history of head traumas? Are they obese?

This is why some people respond to therapies and some people do not. These factors express genes. At times we get sick and don't recover because there are many factors that go into immunity. Prevention is understanding these factors and your genetic expression to plan for health.

Is there a new approach?

As discussed, medicine derives from Newtonian physics since its conception. Medicine observes the body as a bio-machine with specific parts having roles. Each part is broken down into their fundamental mechanical movements. For example, the brain is its bio-computer with thought as a byproduct of the brain's activity. Conventional medical treatment of this bio-machine is through medications and surgery. The goal is to decrease abnormal bio-mechanisms in the physical body.

But what about thoughts and emotions? Can you not love, be disappointed, or frustrated? How does that affect health? Emotions may influence illness through hormonal connections in the brain and body. There's an entire field known as psychoneuroimmunology. This studies on how stress, emotions, and brain functions all interact. Instead of one system and one byproduct, the nervous system, brain, and immune system are acting as one.

Unfortunately, most Americans are on a crash course for disease or degeneration. It can be both physical and emotional.[19]

If someone were to step off a curb at an intersection with a dump truck heading at them, what would you do? You'd like someone to warn you about impending doom so you could make a change and get out of the way.

The problem is the majority of our current medical system is it cannot provide a warning. They measure the damage only after the truck hit you. What's more frustrating is the therapies utilized can create more problems.

My question is, where's the prevention?

For example, when someone has pain in the body, or when a physician is attempting to reduce the pain, the doctor may prescribe Aspirin. There's no doubt Aspirin can reduce pain and increase time needed to form a clot. But it also does much more than the desired lock and key reaction. Aspirin is a group of pharmaceuticals known as non-steroidal anti-inflammatory drugs (NSAIDS). It is well documented that it depletes iron, vitamins K, C, and folate (a vitamin needed to repair blood vessels and makes red blood cells). It hurts kidneys by allowing increased permeability of important kidney cells. Aspirin causes about 3000 deaths from documented cases of abdominal bleeding in the United States per year from normal usage.[20] [21] [22] Tylenol does not have much of an effect on the kidneys, but instead hurts our liver.[23] It slows down required phase I and II of the detoxification process in the liver via the p450 pathway to break it down and neutralize its toxic effects. What's more frustrating is that a simple, useful over the counter medication is easy to buy.

What's more concerning, an individual taking its FDA recommended dosage could die. And this is from using a normal dose, FDA approved, regulated medication. On the flip side, if a natural substance caused over 3000 American deaths per year, we'd have quite a ban on that substance. More likely a massive Federal investigation. Let's take Aspirin one step further. Many patients come into my office because their doctor has told them to take it to prevent a heart attack or cardiovascular event. In 2016, the FDA posted on their website that they have not seen a reduction, or the ability to prevent these issues. [24] [25] [26] [27] Their recommendation is to only use it during or after a cardiovascular event due to the side-effects presented above.

Can you guess how many patients and doctors know this fact? In my experience, it's few. In their defense, how many are looking up products or perusing the FDA website for information?

It is becoming more obvious that pharmaceutical companies are not 100% committed to decreasing disease. They are in business to sell products.

"Many side effects actually cause more disease and increase sales of other products." [28]

The average American is on seven prescriptions. This means if you or someone else is not taking medications, then other Americans are making up the difference. Again, 99% of all pharmaceuticals are not tested with other medications. Or, we rely on China to test them [29] [30] [31] That means there's no real way to find out if there's a counteractive affect whether that's inhibitory or enhancing. It's an educated guess that a patient on X medication prescribed Y medication won't have any side effects or drug interactions. If X medication eliminates a little calcium in the body, and Y medication does the same results as X, there could be issues. These could be as little as cramping, constipation, fatigue, or insomnia.

Or there could be more disastrous effects over time, such as a heart attack or bone loss, causing osteoporosis. Pharmacy is more complicated than the notion of giving this to treat that. Our pharmaceutical industry assumes everyone has the same physiology. It assumes we eat the same, breathe the same air, and work out exactly 60 minutes a day within the correct heart rate zone. This, unfortunately, is fantasy.

It estimated that 10,000 Americans die daily because of these side effects. How is this not our national agenda? Would 10,000 die daily from natural causes and result in a net zero? I haven't found the research to substantiate this possibility. [32] Medicine is the third leading cause of death. [33] [34]Or did those 10,000 people live for five or ten years beyond what they would have lived, only to succumb to the side effects of the therapeutic medication? Was it worth it? It's all relative. If it was pain-free and functioning five years, then why not? If you suffered for those extra five years, then maybe not. I understand these questions are too complex to answer.

Chemistry is more complicated than replacing the substance that you may be missing. Chemistry in your body is not 1+1=2. Many chemical reactions are in fact 1+1= 3 or 8. Or in the case of hormones, neurotransmitters and genes—thousands.

Replacing a substance can have dramatic or detrimental effects. This is why most prescriptions are a trial-and-error basis. How could your doctor know how any substance will affect you? They can't know. And, sometimes your case or conditions take a lot of trial and error.

During my lifetime, I was taught that if you are sick, it is because you must have a genetic defect or an epigenetic expression of the bad genes that are now running your health. Epigenetics are what is happening now. For instance, everyone in your family may have high blood pressure, but you do not. That means you are not expressing the inherited genes. Could you at some point? Sure, but not now.

We understand 90% of American illnesses are lifestyle choices.

This is where we have epigenetic disease expressions. Many food choices affect epigenetic expression for disease. Unfortunately, many of these food choices are generally acceptable to public health officials. Yet, the declining quality of food has enhanced and accelerated common, yet slow, disease processes. It could also be a lack of exercise. Or, a lack of brain stimulation. Or not getting a shoulder, back or neck fixed, allowing inflammation to reside.

Those lifestyle choices contribute to genetic dysfunctions and now epigenetic expression.

There are also non-genetic expressions. For example, say your mother and father bend over daily to lift 200 pounds from the waist. This is the incorrect way to lift and they suffered with back pain their entire adult life. And because you learn from them, as you mature, you'll have back pain too. Is that genetic or a learned behavior?

Here's an interesting phenomenon. In the wild, the wolf and coyote do not have any degenerative diseases such as diabetes, arthritis, gout, or kidney stones. However, once domesticated, our puppy dog friends suffer from the same degenerative disease as their masters. Why? Because of the introduction of disease promoting foods that humans often consume. The foods, medications, and lifestyle choices have the ability to turn on genes that can be responsible for ill health.

If you remember the movie "Twins," Danny Diveto and Arnold Schwartzaneggar were made in a test tube and given the same genetic material. I understand I'm dating myself, but humor me again while I'm making a point. While made in the test tube, which is "In vitro," all the genetic material for size, strength, and looks went to Arnold. Unfortunately, the rest to Danny. I can promise you my genetic output is similar in comparison to Danny.

What I don't want is to have things in my lifestyle that allow the expression of those genes and lay a foundation for disease. So, you can inherit bad or dangerous genes that promote disease. I'm here to explain to you that if you know what those genes are, and you work with someone who can explain the triggers that allow them to express, then you can make the necessary lifestyle and nutritional changes to thwart their progression. I may be biased, but I think that is awesome. We have a choice to change our health and our future if we know how to.

By all probability, I will have Alzheimer's in my lifetime. If I can put that off until my mid 80's, I've won. Why? Because I have all the genes we know today for it, and it is early onset.

What I do understand are the triggers and mechanisms. You can bet your bottom dollar I'm doing all that I can to protect my brain and my body from this debilitating disease. I'm also working on current expression and other potential issues from my inherited DNA.

While you read further, I expect to unlock the full potential of your ability to heal using natural medicine to restore our patients to health. By all probability, you share the same views or are considering learning something new. Many cases do respond to natural medicine. Understand, your cells do have limitations, and there are those who still need conventional medicine. For example, if you smoked for years, your lung cells have changed. They lose their hair and you have a smoker's cough. While certain tissue can heal, the small hairs do not come back like they were before smoking, if ever. You may need medical aids to help you breathe.

WHY YOU NEED TO EDUCATE YOURSELF

My Mentor, Dr. Dowty

Three decades ago Dr. Milton Dowty had a dream to achieve a "No More Excuses" practice. Having been accomplished in music, architectural design, and athletics, he also had a gift for problem solving. He was able to figure out and explain complex situations. Early in his practice, he became fed-up with clinicians having lack of progress. To add insult, he noted increased fees even with a lack of results. And if patients didn't improve, the clinicians made a list of excuses about why an individual was not getting better.

In Dowty's opinion, the status quo was unacceptable.

His unique ability to solve problems came from a fundamental belief for seeking knowledge. If you don't ask the question or find the problem, how do you expect to fix a problem? He then developed a system of nerve-based monitoring that allows doctors to ask the proper questions when testing your body. With this system, he was able achieve his goals of excuse-free patient care.

After 150,000 treatments, Dr. Dowty, a perfectionist, has refined his system so that he can educate doctors. There are portions an individual can use at home without a medical certificate. The body is rather complex, but doesn't have to be so complicated to learn and understand. He wanted his explanations easy enough so everyone could benefit.

During his 44 years as a doctor, he documented conditions that do not require emergency room intervention and had a 92% recovery. Why? The body is frequency-specific with little packets of energy, and Dr. Dowty has translated those frequencies for the benefit of mankind. This system of monitoring the nervous system has been used on over one million individuals. It allows for a complete body assessment, where to treat, what to treat and when to move on. More specifically, which type of tissue to treat and what therapeutic procedures should the doctor use.

In other words, do you use nutrition, body work, balancing, or other therapies? Each therapy aims at the cause of each condition. Being specific reduces the risk of harm and allows for repeatable results.

You are specializing in yourself. You are not only moving a joint, or strengthening a muscle or a ligament. You are fixing the neurological and small packets of energy components of the energetic person you are.

Dr. Dowty understood that treatments for trauma and chronic disease are much too complicated for one specialty to handle. The medical doctor excels in crisis and life-threatening situations. However, there is a huge void between crisis and preventative care. The results are rather low for medical intervention of chronic conditions. Most prevention is after the first symptom, and often that's too late. You know yourself better than anyone else. You can take control of your health by finding where to treat, what to treat, and how to treat.

Before we get into the details of what you can do to help yourself, it is important to understand what we are. Health is not an absence of symptoms. It's a disturbance in those small packets of energy. You can think of these as electrical signals that run the nervous system. It could be large like molecules that get together to signal tissue or cells to allow life to occur. Or it can also be something very small like an electron proton or neutron that is part of an atom. Each has a role in making you who you are. Subtle energy packets and molecules are interconnected within you. And you are connected to those around you. It's important to have a connection to people. Social distancing, though admirable and necessary at times, isn't exactly good for the soul. Humans need to interact and it's more than going online for a webinar or video chat. That's not the same as looking at someone in person. It's touching, feeling, smiling, crying, and being present.

You do not need to understand biochemistry or other medical coursework. Understand that you have an individual bioelectric energy signature. We have many similarities, and genetically speaking, we are about 99.9% the same. It is how we express those genes that has so many variables. My goal is to provide you with the ability to express as you see fit.

From eating, sleeping, exercise, and thinking, each one is a process that undergoes an electromagnetic change. These changes or functions are quantum changes and are essential for life. When there is a disruption, you don't feel well or don't heal. These functions of electromagnetic change occur from subtle energies through subatomic particles. I promised you I won't go into quantum physics or explain Schrodenger's cat. It is part of who we are, so I throw it out there.

CHAPTER 2

Comprehensive Alternative Medicine?

Alternative medicine teaches practitioners there are many factors that can overload your body. These allow disease and body pain to thrive. This is known as inflammation which is a foundation of all disease. When looking at illness and health as multifactorial, you should gain a more effective treatment. The single-cause focus of conventional medicine can often leave too many unanswered questions. You may know what, but how, when, why and what else are punted to a different specialist.

You need to look at the entire body, not just a set of symptoms or a specific condition. In my experience, many medications and prescriptions are treatments for symptomatic relief that can be temporary. Unfortunately, some leave lasting and serious side-effects. They do not focus on the root cause of disease, rather the relief of symptoms. If you're in severe pain and disabled, yes. However, this method is not in the interest or even close to the definition of health.

What's missing is the why. How did you get here? Is it reversible? If not, can we gain function back? Is this medication necessary, and if so, for how long? When do we change if not make improvements in life? Do we monitor with blood tests to make sure we are not causing something else?

Alternative practitioners look at the whole person. They learn to take note of the symptoms, health history, family history, diet, stressors, and triggers. With this information, they hope to discover underlying imbalances such as meridian, stressors, postural, and dietary deficiencies, to name a few.

If your alternative practitioner doesn't take a holistic entire-body approach, they're missing the point as well. If their history is a page that consists of your address, insurance, social security number, and payment information, walk away. Their priority is not your health.

Alternative medicine is not perfect. Sometimes those doctors only pop or crack a neck, have you do some exercises, follow one particular diet, or avoid certain foods. They may even have you take a supplement or do some brain exercises. While these therapies can help, they are also only viewing one system of the multisystemic being you are. How is that any different from conventional medicine?

It isn't that different.

Your doctor needs to do as much as they can, or co-treat with other doctors who can help you in your journey for health with each system for success. Your cause can be very complicated. You may not get to see one doctor, but instead a few. Hopefully, to work together for your benefit. That is easier said than done, but it can work. You need biomechanics and structure work—you need brain work.

As I evolved, my patient load became more and more complex. I haven't had a rolled ankle, knee pain, neck, or lower-back pain as a primary patient for 15 years. Yes, my patients are at times clumsy, and these things come up, but it isn't my day-to-day. We are currently updating our office, and I am taking down all of the certificates and training from the past two decades. Why? Pieces of paper are attempting to define me. I chose to do for my patient what they need and I have a lot of tools. I have yet to have a patient complain about why we aren't learning more and keeping up. I plan to keep it that way.

I understand you could have chemical, electrical, organic, even stress-related causes, or a combination of any of these. In our office, a plan for your recovery and maintenance is created individually for you so that you may function and age at your optimum ability. You deserve that at the very least.

FUNCTIONAL MEDICINE

Functional for the most part means "how" you function. The functional medicine approach is to find an underlying root cause of your condition and get you back to homeostasis, or at least within harmony with your body. This does not mean you have a life-threatening disease, but it could be a chronic disease, or you have been to every doctor without answers. You're sick and tired of being sick and tired.

Functional medicine FM is the application of a detailed history that consists of how, when, where, and why you are seeking help. Things that could contribute to a condition or disease include genetics, lifestyle, or food. History is vital and should be lengthy in your story. Why? What are your triggers? How did you get here? [35]

A (FM) physician should provide a complete physical exam, neurological testing, and most times, blood tests. But FM can look deeper into allergies. Allergies can be environmental, toxins, hormonal, electrical, and many others.

What if you're already diagnosed with a chronic disease such as diabetes, rheumatoid arthritis, or other autoimmune diseases? What can an FM physician do for you? First, one needs to know if they actually have said condition. A series of tests should be run for antibodies both with saliva and blood for tissues for confirmation. Second, once that condition is confirmed, what caused it? Will you need to be with a medical doctor for prescriptions? Or can you dampen the response yourself with a change in diet? Do you also need to work with a holistic practitioner to act as an adjunct therapy to help manage your condition? In some cases, the patient needs medications to function. There could be other conditions or dampen the immune response and teach you the things that add to your inflammation or a medication that depletes your immune system.

If you're autoimmune most of the time, you'll have your autoimmune antibodies for the rest of your life. That said, some patients respond in such a way where they don't look like they ever had a problem to begin with. This is called remission.

Functional medicine doctors, and in my humble opinion, what every doctor's goals should be as a base and then add knowledge and additional tools. Its premise is to restore proper function and balance to your entire body and not focus on one system. FM focuses on identifying and addressing the underlying cause of your illness rather than suppressing the symptoms. This approach, referred to as functional wellness, has enabled FM doctors to help hundreds of patients reverse and heal chronic health issues using a variety of tools, including neurological tests and comprehensive laboratory tests.

An FM doctor assesses your metabolism, hormones, immune system, gastrointestinal system, and nervous system. If they don't create a customized plan to help you regain your health, then don't go back. You are not a cookie-cutter project.

When seeing a functional medicine doctor, they must check your diet, exercise, and lifestyle. Will these need any modifications? Are they working for you? You may need routine laboratory, radiography studies, and even genetics evaluated. I'm not sure how to work without blood tests. Too often there are underlying inflammatory conditions without any symptoms. This is prevention. This is why modern medicine is often failing in the treatment of chronic disease. For many chronic diseases, alternative medicine has success or some benefit. The difference: it involves all aspects of life—the mind, body, and spirit.

Before you run to your nearest FM doctor, I want to make things clear. FM works when used in combination with history, routine testing, and education. There is a caveat. Most FM practitioners take weekend coursework and then a test. These courses are on digestion, detoxification, hormone, immune, cardiovascular, and metabolism conditions. While these are great classes, you are more complicated than a six-weekend course. Some practitioners latch onto one condition. The majority of their patients have: yeast, allergies, parasites, heavy metals, or leaky gut. You could have all or none of them. Then, if dietary or supplements are recommended, you need to understand and test digestion.

Here inlays a problem. If you don't have a functioning nervous system to help you digest, your success rate goes down. Or, all the supplements you take are for not and a complete waste of money. When you don't move efficiently, your systems are going to be under stress. Now, you create inflammation and the higher inflammation you have the shorter a physical treatment will hold. Again, this costs money. In turn, your nervous and digestive systems become inhibited and less efficient. That's why it takes more than six weekends to gain a complete holistic entire-body approach. Using the three pillars of chemistry, movement, and brain function, you can gain an understanding on the how and why and start a plan for recovery.

Traditional medical doctors are not trained for this type of service. In managed care, you most likely have a condition that is affecting more than one of your body's systems. Our medical community specializes in cardiovascular, neurology, rheumatology, gastroenterology, dermatology, and other disciplines. They are trained for acute infection, acute trauma, acute inflammation, and they are best for emergencies. It gets complicated for patients when their condition covers multiple systems. Name a condition that isn't. Chronic conditions go even beyond what is taught in current Functional Medicine classes. There are medical doctors who do learn FM. Great, that's a start, but they need more.

Functional Neurology

Functional Neurology (FN) takes a holistic approach and evaluates for imbalances and disorders in the way the body functions. [36]This is much the same as FM and has the premise of instead of automatically equating certain symptoms with a pathology or disease. FN is a diagnostic representation of your brain and its communication with your nervous system. More exactly, FN works to restore the body's proper neurological functioning without drugs or surgery. This could be the incorporation of brain games, eye movement, and balance. These forms of stimulation are to fire parts of your brain and nervous system with the idea of creating neuroplasticity. That is, new connections to make your brain more efficient. It is the ability of the brain to form and recognize synaptic connections, especially from learning and experience following an injury.

When you learn to play a musical instrument and can play it with your eyes closed, this is neuroplasticity. In our office, we use tools such as measuring your reflex time, balance, memory and other tools that help us understand what we can develop to improve your neuroplasticity.

Consider throwing and catching a ball at age 14 after playing for years verses the same task at the age of 5. You are much better at 14. Why? Neuroplasticity. [37] [38] [39]Yes, you have more neurons at age five. In fact, around 18 months you have the most your will ever have. Just not a lot of connections or plasticity. If you remember the Christmas tree from Charlie Brown, it had thick branches, but no leaves. That's an 18-month-old brain. Move to 35 years old. Now you have climbing ivy for a brain. The branches are not as thick, but they are interconnected and intertwined and quite a tangle. That's neuroplasticity and it can improve at any age.

With FN, it's the communication between different brain regions that can be evaluated. While functional MRI is one of the best tools for observation, there are other tools to evaluate the neuroconnections between different brain regions. For instance, there are different pathways for pain but similar ending points for those pathways. There are different regions for sensations and similar pathways to get to those regions. In simple terms, your brain has backups for when regions or pathways are not working at their optimum.

In a functional MRI, (fMRI) if we could look at the cellular networks, it would look like a bush with a lot of branches and leaves.[40] Conversely, neurodegeneration would look like a tree with a few branches and no leaves. Some forms of neurodegeneration you may have heard of: Alzheimer's, Parkinson's, dementia. So, the denser an fMRI is, the more connections you most likely have. If there is neurodegeneration, it is up to us and your other doctors to discover why and what we can do to mitigate its progression. One of those options is to help generate neuroplasticity by helping you learn new tasks and train other parts to work. In short, use those backup systems if working and make them more efficient. Most of the time, these are tasks you don't like to do or stink at. If in high school math was too hard, and you decided to not do it as an adult, that part of your brain would usually degenerate first. So, guess what your therapy is? Math skills.

If an FN doctor is not doing FM, and vice versa, I don't understand how they expect outcomes. I'm pretty stern on that. If your blood sugar, blood supply, digestion, and oxygen content (often disturbed in anemia) are not normal, then how on earth will your nervous system respond to anything? What if there's a gall bladder issue and you can't absorb fat? This is required for the brain and the central nervous system to buffer electrical signals. For example, most people go to an FN because they have headaches, are dizzy, or had a concussion. Without blood tests, the FN doctor won't be able to adequately predict your outcome. How would an FM doctor know you have trouble in your nervous system, or a signal for digestion, without being an FN doctor? They are embedded together. More importantly, if you have one of the metabolic issues slowing down nerve conduction, such as inflammation, blood sugar imbalances, anemia, or other issues, your brain exercises may fatigue you too quick and you might actually get worse! If your FM doctor isn't checking you for digestion, then all those supplements could be a massive waste of money. The reality is not a lot of doctors integrate the two schools of thought. But isn't that the issue with modern medicine? It matters for all doctors regarding this—integration and system overview are paramount to your health.

I'm not a fan of being pigeonholed as a functional medicine doctor, functional neurologist, sports doctor, nutritionist, acupuncturist, or by any other coursework I have completed. My license is that of a chiropractor. I happen to do so much more. I spent over $1,000,000 on my education above current chiropractic tuition. Yuck! I found early what motivates my continued learning: knowing that not all patients would respond to a treatment. Or, some even stop responding. There's a big Why in there. Some would respond to exercise, others dietary changes. For some, they needed acupuncture, and from blood tests a plan to be well or dietary changes. Almost everyone needed at least one supplement. I use supplements to support or fix an issue we find in blood or urine testing. I do not believe or find clinically you can supplement yourself out of a disease condition. It's more complicated than taking a pill.

According to Einstein, matter is defined as stored energy. As you sit reading this, you are metabolizing and creating energy. This energy is not even close from what is stored. Think of yourself as a night log for a campfire, not to be morbid or obtuse. To the touch, you're cooler on the outside. You don't feel more than 100 degrees and don't seem to be metabolizing much when compared to other mammals who are quite warm to the touch. Likewise, a piece of wood is cool to the touch. However, once wood—or more morbidly, flesh—is placed on fire, an enormous amount of energy is released that was once stored. Energy is stored in matter.

While science becomes more sophisticated every year, scientists still look at the world in simple terms. You are a bio-machine that has interchangeable parts. Surgeons are hands down the best bio-machine mechanics, each year getting more and more micro as techniques evolve. One could consider orthopedics surgeons the carpenters, vascular surgeons the plumbers. This does not explore the reason for the problem, but instead is part specific.

Where is the holistic approach in this? Where do prayer, nutrition, lifestyle, and thoughts fall into medicine, a placebo? Again, has no one ever become better because they thought they could or someone prayed for them? I know many who have overcome conditions because they believed they would. How can this not be a valid function?

If you look at FDA requirements, the way a medication is approved is that it must beat the placebo effect, and by a very small amount. In the case of anxiety and anti-depressants, the standard is less than one percent. That means there's a chance for FDA-approved medications to be circulating that only inched out a better outcome than a placebo.[41] [42] [43] There are those who thought they were receiving said drug but did not. Keep in mind those with placebo can think and perceive side effects even though they never received the drug.

Who knew we could actually think ourselves well or sick?

The study of molecular biology consists of a lock and key concept and was my first degree. This would mean if you knew the specific molecular cause, then medicine should be a fail-safe. In many diseases, every molecular option is not completely understood. I get there have been advances. It's fascinating to understand how the immune and nervous systems communicate through molecular signals. Or, to test how they work. But it's not absolute. There are other ways for your body to communicate and function.

This is what drew me toward my second degree in this field. If I could understand the mechanisms, the pathways then I could be a better student, runner, future doctor. Fast forward a few years. If the mechanistic lock-and-key model worked, then anyone exposed to the flu virus this year will get it, period. Why do some people get sick and others do not when exposed? Is it because one has a better lock? There are too many factors to be exact on how we get sick and how we stay healthy.

Most aspects of medicine and in our Westernized viewpoint lack an appreciation or devalues intangible things. These include emotions, body-mind-spirit, life force, and the subtle energies of the test subject. An emotional patient who has anxiety or depression tends to be prescribed medication. This approach is a lock-and-key neurotransmitter-based prescription in lieu of attempting to understand the bigger picture of human dynamics. We are multidimensional complex bundles of energy. There are other parts of you then prescribing your body neurotransmitters. How is your digestion, your memory, your energy? Is your blood sugar handling perfectly? How does that medication get absorbed? Detoxified? Metabolized? Do your joints function and how is your blood supply? Should those with anxiety also find a cardiologist, endocrinologist, neurologist, rheumatologist, gastroenterologist, orthopedist? Technically, yes. You are defined by more than one system and they are all working together to make you function.

Modern science is often missing the point of what is their foundation of higher learning. Science is by definition the expression of the vibratory frequencies that creates the structure of our universe. That in itself is very exciting because it provides the groundwork for understanding. By defining science, it is probable if we are not looking at humans and their health as vibration frequencies. And if we are not, then there is a chance we are looking at it all wrong.

Medical doctors at times are too quick to raise a disbelieving eyebrow to older approaches. Instead they chose newer medications that have similar functions to natural methods. These natural options could be herbals, plants, and homeopathy that have been used to heal humans since the beginning of time. Granted, some older ideas have been researched and do not have any use. That said, it doesn't make sense to me as so many pharmaceuticals are often refined natural therapies.

My point is, we are more than biological machines, as medicine portrays. Herbs and homeopathics are at root, energy. Yes, they do have proteins, fats, and carbohydrates which are lock and key. But they also contain a frequency. These frequencies work on a different vibration then medicine or matter. But if you didn't know it, medications are vibrational too. They have a vibration that allows the subtle energies of the body to accept them and achieve a desired result.

Consider this: if medications were vitally important to sustain life, wouldn't they grow somewhere?

This is not a slam against the pharmacy world, as they do great things through medications to stave off death. It is only a question of man versus nature; who is more insightful? Has anyone become better or worse because they believed they would? Has anyone responded to prayer, lifestyle changes and no medical intervention? Or are we all doomed unless we agree to full medical advice?

I tend to believe it is a little bit of both. Some natural remedies are debunked for the claims made. Ok, I'll allow it because it's true. But in contrast, hundreds of medications are now used for effects they were not originally intended for. Viagra and methotrexate come to mind. Viagra was formulated for high blood pressure and had secondary uses for erectile dysfunction. Methotrexate was a chemotherapy agent that is now used for rheumatoid arthritis and other autoimmune inflammatory conditions. There has to be some level of openness that one side or the other is not utilitarian or always right, and there is a need for both at times. In my biased opinion, we should do our best to function as natural as possible, because medications are man-made and not as perfect as nature.

When it comes to vibrational therapy, we all vibrate with different degrees. Those in harmony are well; those out of tune are prone to illness and disease. Remember Psychoneuroimmunology (PNI)? PNI investigates the connection of thoughts, emotions and the actual physiological events that evolve following those non-physical events. [44] If we have more stress that we perceive, then we will put out more stress hormones and age faster. This reduces repair and immunity. Yet, another individual in the same stressors may have little to no adverse effects. Why? Again, we have different unique biochemistry. The most important concept is that we have different vibrations.

To be more scientific, there are many opportunities for vibration proof of how we exist and what is affecting us. Here are some basic examples we are all familiar with. Sounds waves vibrate and do not have any physical matter, it is only energy. They can be very destructive under high amplitude such as in the case of an earthquake or tsunami. An X-ray is energy passing through an object. Televisions and radios have receivers for transmission of electronic radio waves. There are cosmic waves such as ultraviolet light, gamma rays, and electromagnetic frequencies (EMF). Lightning, thunder, ultrasound and sonar waves, microwaves, and WIFI vibrate as energy we can see and/or use.

In medicine, an EKG is necessary to test vibrating electronic waves from the heart. This shows proof of a previous heart attack, not to predict the future. The vibration or electronic signature only changes after the fact, it's not prevention in the case of an EKG. My cell phone vibrates, accepts cellular frequencies and is now connected to my watch. My updated watch now monitors electrical vibrations of my heart. It knows that it's me on my phone and what application I wish to open because I touch my screen and it reads by biometrics. Chances are you've exposed to vibrational energy, and we can move on to deeper topics.

CHAPTER 3

How To Communicate With Your Doctor

Often, I have been asked by my patients, "What should I ask the doctor I'm being referred to?" Or I'm told, "I don't know what to ask."

I have attempted to recreate many questions I would ask in an office or hospital setting. Also, to provide a reasonable step-by-step direction so that you and your doctor can communicate. This is to help you have the best opportunity for success for you or your loved ones.

Many of my patients provide feedback and say they felt the previous doctor wasn't listening, that they attempted to tell their story only to be interrupted with a series of standard checklist questions. Have you ever felt ignored in a physician's office and left wondering why you ever visited their office in the first place? I have. For the most part, four times out of five, your diagnosis is made on your history. Yet, in my experience, doctors are listening less and less. They're required to ask a series of questions. They now have limited time and are forced by insurance contracts to see more and more patients per day. These insurance reimbursement cuts and other limitations decrease your doctor's opportunity to provide a thorough examination.[45]

Why do doctors test?

I for one am not a savant or clairvoyant. At times I like to think I know what I'm talking about. But after an examination, a complete review of history, and testing, I still am surprised from time to time on the condition that someone is indeed living. The results from laboratory testing may be essential for detection and management for many conditions. They are practical aiding in the early diagnosis of a particular disorder before the obvious signs and symptoms appear. If you can't find it, often you can't treat it.

Also, it can help find the cause of a condition. This can rule in or out other diagnoses or disorders that cannot be ruled out from just a physical examination and the severity of said condition. Furthermore, early recognition of those patients allows a doctor in our managed health care system to refer to the appropriate specialist. The purpose of testing is to reduce health care costs by reducing guessing. Then, with that information, be able to track the effectiveness of a therapy. Through this, the patient and doctor gain motivation through feedback.

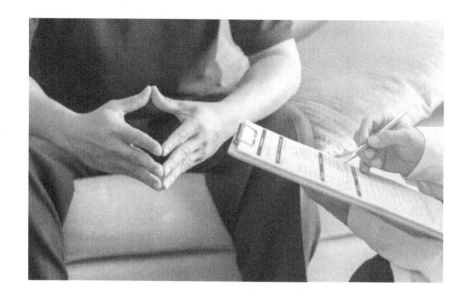

In my humble opinion, the bottom line is we are all different through the way we eat, think, live, and work. Although there are critical numbers that are truly not compatible with life, there are many factors that come into play with the health of an individual. For instance, toxins, drugs, inhalants, chemicals, allergies, even vitamins and minerals can cause a change in a test. Any can lead to some of them being false positives or false negatives. When a patient comes into my office and we run a stool sample test called an occult blood or guaiac test. If they are self-medicating with Vitamin C, it will show up positive on the test, even if they don't have any blood in their stool. Hence, physicians and their patients need to understand specificity and sensitivity for laboratory testing. Specificity is whether or not if we can find what we are looking for and you are correct for both positive and negative results. And sensitivity is how many times out of a 100 can we detect it. Both a vital to any testing and your doctor must know these outcomes and if future or repeat testing is warranted.

Many illnesses and causes of death are well-documented to be the results of substandard health habits such as excess fat, excess sugar intake, alcohol, lack of regular exercise, tobacco use, and obesity. If you're a physician who isn't testing your Body Mass Index (BMI) on a regular basis, then you're missing out. A healthy BMI is below 25. Overweight is 25-29.9 and over 30 is obese.

BMI is important to check because the blood chemistries as a whole trend outside the reference range of "normal" as the BMI goes up. This is why diabetes leads to cardiovascular disease and events such as heart attacks and strokes. This is why it is important to know what your values are and how you can make them better.

For the most part, most American's don't know that you can reverse heart disease and type II diabetes by following one or several natural protocols. One of these "natural" methods has been clinically tested for over 25 years by an endocrinologist. This doctor hasn't had to refer one of his patients to the emergency room, a common side effect of diabetes and cardiovascular disease. Instead, his office uses a protein molecule where its researcher was awarded the Nobel Prize in medicine in 1998.

Why aren't we all using this or something similar? Because this is too simple. That, and natural proteins don't generate much revenue.

We're taught that cholesterol is bad. It was a total mistake by God or the universe to put it in your body. Cholesterol is the evil that keeps Americans fat, sick, and poor. I'll pile on a little bit more to the nonsense we've been educated over the past 40 years. The American Diabetic and the American Cardiology Associations have dietary recommendations that are absurd. They both suggest even if you are diabetic, eating a low-fat, whole grain "sugar" diet is heart healthy when in fact, it promotes the disease. There are thousands of research articles disputing this claim. Whole grain affects insulin, a hormone vital to both diabetics and cardiovascular patients. Cholesterol is actually a good thing. It's in every single cell in your body. It is necessary for brain function. So, we can't get rid of all of it. There are many types of cholesterol, and from what we're taught, the Low Density Lipoprotein (LDL) or "evil" cholesterol is a killer.

However, there are two types of LDL that indicate disease, and one that if it isn't present in our cell walls, the cell dies. Therefore, the type of LDL is important. On the flip side, we are taught High

Density Cholesterol (HDL) is considered "good." Again, there are currently three known types of HDL of which two are cardiovascular healthy and one is not. I'm not out to confuse you, but instead get you to ask for adequate testing. Simply testing total cholesterol or a lipid panel with HDL, LDL, total cholesterol and triglycerides is a far cry from adequate. This type of testing is the equivalent of taking your car to the mechanic and they walk around it and tell you what's wrong when you have engine trouble.

This is why new patients of mine who didn't take much stock in health present with good HDL numbers. But when we run the fractionalized test to split the different types of LDL and HDL it actually shows the bad HDL present.[46] I guess you could say it gives folks a false sense of health security. Yet, this is the foundation of our health care system. Also, life insurance only looks at total numbers. Once these new patients wanting help with their health see the "true" cholesterol numbers they awake to the truth. They tend to realize that sugar for breakfast, soda for fluid intake, and pasta for dinner doesn't make them "healthy" and a good HDL isn't what they thought.

My purpose is to inform you on what you can do for you and your family. Every health-based decision is yours and as doctors we can only recommend and tell you what our opinions are. We can give you the pros and cons of any test or procedure and we can even try to scare you into something, although I am a firm believer that is unethical. If you recall the Hippocratic Oath, "First, do no harm." That is where we should start. I encourage you to learn as much as you can, as in the end, you are the best doctor for you.

Your physician's recommendation and clinical experience play a big part, but you alone have the ability to say "yes", and at times, "no." From a conventional MD to a functional medicine doctor, they may see things different from one another. But the fact of the matter is the numbers are the same. If you've ever played chess at a high level, there are methods to learning. A chess instructor may explain to you that if you are stuck, stand up and look at the board in a different way. The pieces are still the same, it's a different point of view and can reveal things that aren't clear even to the educated and well-trained eye.

Eighty percent of the money consumed in our country for health care is spent on chronic degenerative diseases. [47] [48] You have heard of these names. Cardiovascular disease, diabetes, cancer, kidney failure, and arthritis. For the most part, these are preventable with proper lifestyle changes. Note I did not say DIET. If you go on a diet, you'll most likely go back to your old habits. It is my opinion a poor diet promotes disease and thus premature death. I'll hammer down dietary intake later because it is an important pillar.

Sometimes we need a good kick in the rear to get motivated. By understanding what you can do this will get you moving towards a better quality of health. Did you know that close to twenty percent of Americans are afraid to go to the doctor although they feel "okay"? And sixty percent would rather change their diet than take medication. This trend has been going on for 20 years, but are we as a whole doing it? Well, sometimes. Maybe. You eat healthy or consider health outside of the holiday season. And not during the NCAA basketball tournament or Superbowl. And oh yeah, the 4th of July, your birthday, vacation, office parties, etc.

Ah ha! We justify. Eighty-seven percent of Americans recognize the importance of exercise, so we're not ignorant.[49] [50] [51] But less than half of us walk even three miles a week. Is it that hard or asking too much? Ask someone who has a chronic disease and they'll tell you absolutely it's that hard! If you're a chronic person, my goal as a doctor is to get you better. If you're not chronic, I want you to learn as much as you can so that you don't. I can assure you being chronic is not a quality life. Remember, most of these are preventable, so let's focus to prevent. When it comes down to it, if you don't do something about it now, when will you? And with declining insurance benefits, you will be required to spend your personal funds on your health. Should you wait until you are sick or chronic, you will end up spending a lot more in managing your condition. A chronic condition that will take away from so many things you want to accomplish in life. More importantly, how you desire to live.

Your plan for treatment should be explained to you. Sometimes your physician is ordering tests to make a proper diagnosis. You may need to come back for further answers and sometimes further testing. Once it's understood what your problem is, you should have a plan on how to treat, if it is fixable, or if it needs to be managed.

In any office there should be informed consent. This is education on what will happen if you do nothing, or wait for treatment, alternative options, and discussion on any future procedures and tests you may need to have. Informed consent is much more than saying, "Let's do this procedure and see what happens."

It's also good to get to know a bit more about your doctor, their philosophy, and experiences. Would you go to a pediatrician who detests children? They exist. How about a chiropractor or nutritionist who knows and says all the right things but smokes and eats fast food at lunch?

If there's a procedure or surgery, make sure that you understand the setting. Are you the first procedure of the day, or the last, when your doctor is tired? Ask your doctor how they get along with the staff. Do they have good rapport with the anesthesiologist, if needed? I've seen a surgeon fight with an anesthesiologist on occasion, and I wouldn't want that during my surgery. Also, ask, "How many procedures have you performed? I don't want to be your first."

Your records are your property. Unfortunately, now they are the government's property as well. In the future I expect us to have a health score that acts much like a credit score.

The worse your score is, the more you will pay for and be responsible for your health. As insurance regulations can no longer omit pre-existing conditions, they will find ways to charge you for many conditions, and more so if you created it through a lack of self-preservation.

When you don't take care of yourself or have unhealthy habits, it costs you in the workplace. For the past decade, insurance carriers at large companies have been testing not only for drugs, but nicotine from tobacco products in your blood and urine. If you pass, you get a deduction in your health care costs. If you don't, you get to pay the most.

At times, you will have to pay for your records for any doctor's office. I suggest when you get your notes and any copies of tests, you keep a file in a safe place at home, if not scanned on PDF. I can't tell you how helpful it is for me as a physician to see a few years of notes, tests, and procedures to get an idea of how a patient has been treated and tested. Also, to see what hasn't been examined or ruled out and not repeat things that are not necessary.

Managed care makes it harder and harder to see a specialist. Often, when I must refer, it's months, if not closer to a year, to get a patient in who isn't terminal but clearly needs medical help. Depending on your insurance carrier, you may have to go to one or two doctors just to get to where you need to be. Who is supposed to take the history, do an exam, run tests? Insurance may limit how many tests are done per year, regardless who runs them. Doctors are becoming more frustrated with regulation and many just want the time to help their patients. Furthermore, over the past decade, research is finding physicians are paying too much attention to their electronic devices and not enough to their actual patients, so much so that it's hindering doctors' ability to do their jobs.

Older physicians believe that some doctors are losing the old skills that are critical to making a quick and accurate diagnosis. These skills tend to be part of the physical exam. This part of an appointment is when a doctor uses touch, sight, and all the other senses to learn about what's ailing the patient. You may recall flashing a light into your pupils, being observed how you walk, tapping on your abdomen, and your doctor listening to your chest with a stethoscope. These are essential skills. A doctor is to look, touch, listen, and rebound.

Today's modern physician now relies more on data than anything else. If you have a new headache, you get to help pay for an MRI and a neurological consult, if not a cardiology consult and muscle relaxers, or something close. Blood tests are then ordered for future information. The doctor's focus has gone away from the patient, their history and their story, and quickly their focus is on diagnostics.

I am a firm believer you must be touched. You need a real exam. Someone needs to inspect you, check for subtle hints or clues. More important, a thorough history. My intake is 38 pages and I ask you to write me a story about your life health. Why? Clues.

For example, a patient presents with memory lapses. Off to the MRI, right? Hold on a minute. How long have they had these? Fifty years or five days? One of those requires an MRI and the other does not. I have hundreds of stories where patients had growths, pain, and other discomforts and were not touched. How can you do that? Is there an ESP exam that I've been sheltered from? Because if there is, I want in. We spend somewhere between 1 1/2 - 2 hours on our initial history and exam and that would save time. We do this to narrow our focus, especially in complex cases, which most are.

I recently had a patient come in with abdominal pain. Her last doctor had diagnosed her with endometriosis and ovarian cysts. After reading her history and looking under the surgery section, she had a complete hysterectomy 15 years ago. Therefore, there was no uterus or ovaries to treat. How frustrating! I see this from all types of doctors and alternative doctors. I may sound like a broken record. If your intake form is your name, insurance card, and address I would recommend someone else. I promise you, that is not how that doctor, of any type, was taught or what is required to perform.

CHAPTER 4

Physical Exam and Blood Tests

In general, a physical exam consists of several different tests based on your presentation. But there are a few things that are a must. If they are not present, you should insist on receiving them from your physician. Otherwise they cannot confirm your symptoms or order the proper tests.

Doctors are getting more pressure to perform better with limited time from insurance companies or know about every single disease, medication, treatment, and protocol. It's an impossible feat both the media and pharmaceutical industry has placed on doctors through advertisements.[52]

You can't know everything. Below are the bare basics you deserve in an office setting. I'm providing you the details in how we were all taught and why we were to do it that way.

General overview

Your doctor or their staff should be observing you upon arrival. How you walk, talk, and communicate is important. Do you have an even head carriage, shoulders, and gait? Are you able to sit up? Can you sit comfortably? Are you breathing without difficulty? Did you arrive on time or late? How is your handwriting? Can you follow directions? Was it difficult or stressful to get to their office?

These observations provide your doctor with the ability to decipher where they need to focus. I had a patient walk into my office once looking for a cure for toenail fungus who arrived 90 minutes early because they got lost easily and had been in four fender benders that month. They clearly had more than a fungal issue, and we immediately started with brain function testing and blood supply.

Blood Pressure

We all know about blood pressure. I don't place a ton of stock in blood pressure because someone can be nervous or have had a bad day. They could have had someone cut them off while driving on the way to the office. And there are other sources that change blood pressure including food and medications.

Blood pressure should be taken on both arms. Blood pressure is the initial way to find out if there's a blood supply problem. If the top number (systolic) is twenty points or more than the bottom number (diastolic), this is the first indicator that something is off. So, insist on taking it on both arms. Is it the same in both? What if it isn't? If the "good" side is the only one tested, then you may miss the "bad" or diseased side.

It's your health and it doesn't take that long to get it right. Also, posture is important as well. Are you standing, sitting, or laying down when the blood pressure is taken? Those should all be close and there are guidelines for these positions. Again, if there's a big difference in blood pressure then this could state a blood pressure, or as I like to explain, a blood supply problem. I then begin running cardiovascular testing or refer to a specialist.

Looking in Eyes and Ears

When your doctor pulls out their device to look into your eyes, they use an ophthalmoscope. And for your ears, an otoscope. These very important instruments allow the doctor to view internal working of your body without cutting you open. While looking in the ear, your doctor is looking for any color change. The color of your tympanic membrane (ear drum), swelling, infection, presence of foreign bodies or fluid helps assess ear health. Your ear should be pulled back and the doctor's hand with the instrument should be placed against or close to your chin to allow proper viewing. Something I've witnessed often is improper use of the instrument and incorrect placement. That may not give the physician the best impression, or they may not be able to see what they need to see. Before your doctor is inserting the otoscope, they should observe the outside of your ear and if the entrance to the auditory canal is normal in appearance.

When your doctor looks in your eyes, they are actually looking first at your artery and veins. This is the only place in your body we can see your vascular system and get an idea what your health is. Of course, cataracts and other ocular disturbances can be investigated here or lead to further testing. Your doctor is looking to see if your eyes are round, regular, and equal. Do you react to light, can you see all fields, and do your eyes move to all fields? Is there any abnormal movement or flickering of the eyes or eyelids?

You should also take a minute to view an eye chart to see if your vision is declining or remaining stable. Also, you should be tested for color recognition. Colors should be the same in brightness from left to right to determine eye function. This also evaluates the occipital lobe of your brain for inflammation or degeneration.

Hearing

A tuning fork or sound device may also be used to briefly evaluate auditory perceptions. If they are found, further investigation with an audiologist to assess auditory function is your next step. You should be able to hear the tuning fork at the top of your head equal from left to right. You should also hear it easier when testing each side when placed in front of your ear than on the bone behind it. This is the difference between air and bone conduction. If you cannot hear air more than bone, it is abnormal. Your doctor needs to observe if your ear canal is red. This could state inflammation that could be local or even food allergies. Your ear is connected by the eustachian tube to the gastrointestinal tract. That means allergies in the digestive system, respiratory, and nasal cavity can all affect your hearing.

Vibration

A tuning fork is a wonderful way to assess nervous system function from hearing to swelling in the sinuses by placing it on the forehead. Or one could place it on the body in different ways and see if you feel vibration. Then compare left and right sides. This vibration test is a neurological test for the parietal lobe of your brain, and part of its function is to feel vibration.

Say Ahh

Looking in the mouth is another good way to assess health. Those with periodontal gum disease are at higher risk for diabetes, heart disease, and other chronic diseases. Can you swallow? What do your tonsils look like, healthy or infected? Does your tongue move? What do the veins look like under your tongue? Is the tongue pink? Or is it coated? If it is, what color?

Any of these visual findings led to more tests and questions. Can you open your mouth with the same left and right motion? What is the color of your lips, tongue, tonsils, mucosa, and pharynx? How is the saliva on the teeth, under the tongue, into the back of the mouth? Your saliva is very important to observe. This is where digestion begins. If you have IBS, IBC, bloating, indigestion, diarrhea, heartburn or many others, saliva tells your doctor a story. I can't tell you how many times this is where I started our treatment protocols when no one else looked.

Lymph Nodes and Thyroid examination

Lymph nodes in your neck, arm pits, and groin should also be examined. If you're also getting a breast exam, the lymphatics need to be examined all the way to your elbow. That may also be the case if you have a cold or upper respiratory condition.

80

Lymph nodes of your neck should be investigated with you looking forward and to the side as well as under the chin. Missing any of these are a mistake. Are they normal size, and do they move? If it is tender or painful, you need to let your doctor know. Your thyroid should be examined for swelling or changes. Sometimes your doctor will have you swallow to get an idea where your neck cartilage is and then palpate your thyroid. They are looking for swelling and specific to the thyroid, nodules. If you have any of those, a diagnostic ultrasound will be ordered. For both thyroid and lymph nodes, if nodules are found and there is no explanation through symptoms or blood tests, I will inform you to expect a biopsy. This is where the node or thyroid nodule is excised (cut out) and then sent to a pathologist to see why it is that size. If it is from your thyroid, 95% of all nodules are benign.[53]

Pulses x 12

Pulses need to be felt, not only in your wrist but at the elbow, groin, knee, ankle, and foot. There are twelve spots to examine. Often, we find vascular problems from left to right or upper extremity, or lower extremity on this simple test alone. In a chart, these are graded from I-IV with II being the normal.

Reflexes—everyone has had their knee hit with a reflex hammer. Do you know that only gives you one nerve test? How many nerves do you have in your body? There are other tests behind the foot, the wrist, and both sides of the elbow. It takes eight seconds to test all these and it gives so much information on your health. Your doctor can use a reflex hammer on all your digits and most muscles. So, if you have a weak side or extremity, it is not uncommon to have multiple sites of reflexes to see what is working proper and what is not.

Muscle Testing

Muscle Strength is not a measure of strength to see if you or the doctor is stronger, but a series of about six major muscle groups. Each is tested on both sides of the body to see if you can contract. This assesses what is called alpha motor neuron. When a push or pull is placed into a joint, can the associated muscles react? If so, the muscle and nerve are intact. If not, they need to be investigated or tested more. Strength is graded 1-5 with five being normal and full function. Muscles are also evaluated for any abnormal appearance, such as in a tear, is there any tenderness? Do they have heat or loss of muscle, atrophy? Any one of these should lead to further investigation of "why." And once that is understood, how bad is it? What needs to be treated, if anything, to get it back to proper function?

Listening To Your Heart, Lungs, and Other Parts

Heart and Lungs Auscultation. This is the part where the stethoscope is in use and no one should be talking. When listening to the heart, there are four areas to check. These four areas begin with one on your right side close to where your breastbone and collarbone meet, then to the left side, then on the left at the bottom of the rib cage, and then about 4-6 inches out from there. This allows the physician to check the chambers and valves of the heart for normal sounds.

Depending on the type of stethoscope your doctor may be able to record heart sounds for replay or send to a specialist.

Your doctor should also listen to the carotid arteries in the neck, especially if you have, or your family has, or if you may possibly have any cardiovascular disease. Any findings would warrant a carotid ultrasound to check blood flow from your heart to your brain.

Before anyone touches your abdomen, your physician should listen to you first. If not, this could change the bowel sounds and give a different clinical picture then if not touched. Also, your abdomen is divided medically into four quadrants. Each quadrant should be listened to for any abnormal sounds. Your physician will also palpate your abdomen. They are looking for any masses, tenderness, hernias, abdominal aneurysms, or rigidity. Also feeling for bowel, liver, and spleen swelling.

The doctor should listen to four areas on your lungs, two front and two back, with you taking a deep breath. They may also ask you to say "ninety-nine" or another word for the assessment of fluid. Sometimes it requires a few more depending on what the physician is hearing or looking for. In addition, you may have to blow into a device called a spirometer. This device measures how much air you can get into and out of your lungs and the speed of inhale and exhale. Last, your doctor may measure around your chest before and after a deep breath with a tape measure. In a perfect world, you would get all three, especially if you had a lung or respiratory condition.

Weight, Body Fat, and BMI

Body fat and body mass index (BMI) are a vital test to assess your health and recovery. First, body fat can discover metabolic disorders. The most important is BMI. In a perfect world you'll be under 25. Over 25-29 is considered overweight, and above 30 is obese. Once above 25, your risk for chronic diseases are heightened.[54]

BMI isn't a perfect system. If you have a body builder at five feet tall, they are obese on these charts. Also, an overweight person at 6'6" doesn't show up obese, but instead, normal. BMI is more for the general masses. I prefer body fat. The best test is when you get tested underwater but it's tested almost exclusively at colleges. So, you can get an electrical impedance device that you either stand on barefoot, or hold out with your hands. You input your height, weight, age and body type. There's a 5-10% error with these devices, but they are immediate and you can track any changes. Of course, it's different for children. [55]

Of course, weight can change with fluctuations from many factors. We all know avoiding regular exercise and overeating are two major causes. When should your weight be measured? Often, yet consistent. This means it doesn't have to be done daily, but at the same time of day. Best is in the morning after voiding and before eating. This keeps the test, the scale, consistent. Changes of more than 10 pounds in a month without a discerning reason are red flags. Make sure and tell your doctor about these if you find them at home.

Gait, Walking, Balance

The fastest way to aging is not being able to balance. When is the last time you were checked? Can you walk on your toes, heels, balance on one foot? Loss of balance and coordination decrease your body's ability to recover, repair, and lessens immunity.

Balance testing and gait evaluation help your doctor know how your brain is communicating with your body. Currently, I run upwards of forty different brain tests. Can you remember words in a few minutes, thirty minutes? Can you state five words beginning with the same letter? Can you move your hands rapidly, and is it the same on both sides? How do your fingers move? Together or separately? Can you put one foot in front of the other and balance? Can you do it with your eyes closed?

If you've ever seen a sobriety test, the police have their suspects walking and balancing, touching their nose and reciting numbers while walking.[56] It's a test for an anterior cerebellum. There are many inflammatory processes that affect all parts of the cerebellum.

The number one suspect is gluten. Yep, you look drunk with gluten ataxia.[57 58 59 60 61]

We encourage everyone to record themselves walking. Do both arms swing? Do you walk like a toddler? Do you look like you just got off a cattle drive? Does your head move? Or do you lean forward and shuffle? These are all diagnostic. Also, if you record yourself over time, you will be able to document changes. Balance and how you walk are instrumental in early diagnosis of brain inflammation and neurodegeneration.[62 63]

Orthopedics

When you have joint pain, you will often be tested with an orthopedic test. Sometimes these check for joint integrity, ligament laxity, or other losses. Depending on the movement of a joint or the pressing into an area, your doctor may look a little deeper. Also, sensation with or without pain gives the physician a clinical picture of what is the problem. Your doctor can then decide from the test what needs to be done. This could be conservative such as ice or immobilization, or mobile such as chiropractic, physical therapy, acupuncture, or injections. Or if you are with intense pain or had a poor orthopedic test. You may need an immediate image test and bracing.

Skin Deep

Your physician should make some general observations such as looking at your skin evaluating for lesions, abrasions, moles, color changes and anything else out of the normal. If you have a mole or skin change, when did it occur? What is your lifestyle, family history? Will you need a biopsy or can it wait? I encourage everyone to take a picture. If you can't get into your doctor immediately, then you can provide a timeline with pictures of a suspect area. Again, no change in three months, not that aggressive. If you can see change in three weeks, then that will get your doctor's attention.

Female Exam

For a female exam there are several processes. First, the breast exam. It is ideal to do these at home and should you find an inconsistent issue you can discuss with your doctor. I will walk you through the correct breast exam your doctor should use. But you should be doing these at home and you can do what your doctor does for you in your in-home breast exam.

You should be observed with your arms down and up. Your doctor will be looking for changes in breast contour. And if one or both breasts have normal movement with your arms, or if something is adhered to the thoracic wall. Sometimes for further investigation you may be bent over with arms up and down. Once the physical breast exam begins your doctor should touch on the outside of the breast first light with tiny circles ending at the nipple. A second time will be deeper, both feeling for any abnormalities. The nipple should not be touched but instead pressed on the side of the breast looking for abnormal discharge.

During a pelvic exam, no doctor should ever tell you they are going to "put" anything in you. That's unprofessional. For starters, there needs to be a visual inspection. Yes, you can have lesions and infections on the outside of the skin. Then a physical exam of the labial folds and anus to rule out other lesions or hemorrhoids. A speculum is a tool that when used expands the inside of the vaginal wall so the doctor can better view your cervix. The best ones have a light source for better viewing and this is when a Pap smear test is performed. After the Pap, a physical exam for ovaries and uterus dysfunction will complete your exam. Every woman is different on how they feel comfortable in receiving a pelvic exam. Ask around. If you like conversation or total silence, the word on those doctors exists. Most women have told me they prefer hearing their doctor walking them through each part of the procedure because it feels more professional. Let your doctor know how you prefer to be treated. Last, if you are uncomfortable with a male or female doctor, make sure that before you make an appointment who will be performing the exam. Sometimes it's the doctor's assistant or nurse practitioner for a pelvic exam or even another doctor whom you may not know. If the incorrect person comes in, speak up.

Male Exam

If you are a male, your physician should inspect and then squeeze your penis down looking for any discharge. Your inguinal nodes will then be evaluated about half way down your leg. Your testicles will be palpated for any nodules as well as structures known as the epididymis and spermatic cord. You should be checking your testicles at home for nodules or painful areas every month. Following that an, insert a finger below your testicles into the pelvic cavity to perform a hernia test.

Then you should be evaluated for prostate health. You will be placed on your side or asked to bend over while your doctor feels your prostate for swelling, lumps or inflammation. Should something be out of the ordinary, expect a biopsy with blood tests.

I've had more than one man suggest or seek small-stature and petite urologists because they have smaller hands. This is nonsense. But let me make it easier to understand. I have short stubby hands. I cannot always feel the entirety of a prostate when I performed them. So, if you have issues and the doctor cannot perform the digital exam, you are headed for a biopsy. Choose who you want. I recommend someone who can perform the test and examine you for function.

Who to choose?

After 20 years, I have wondered if I should change my practice name to: "The Best Lab Test for You." I bring this up because so many doctors who are alternative, or moving from medical to alternative, have a lot of misinformation on the validity and application of blood tests. Don't get me wrong. I've taken the majority of those courses, and for the most part, considered using those tests until I gathered the necessary information.

No doctor can be everything for every patient. But we can do many things to provide the best treatment and testing options available. It is our duty as doctors to understand the sensitivity and specificity for any test ordered. And how each impacts the outcome or updates to your treatment plan.

When I was in training, my mentor made me run every test on myself before ordering the same for a patient. Otherwise, how can you explain a procedure? My years in clinical pathology have served me well. I vet each lab we work with for proof of testing and evidence of medical approval.

In the two months before the Covid pandemic, our new patients and out-of-town patients were bringing in lab test results to start the new year. It's disheartening to explain to a patient that their doctor(s) didn't understand the ordered test. Let me explain.

There are a lot of companies testing for food allergies, intestinal barriers, heavy metals, parasites, hormones, and genetics. Not all these companies have FDA or CMS approval. While most people are familiar with the FDA, you may not be with CMS. CMS is a government institute that assures testing validity, efficacy, and whether a test should, or should not be approved for payment. If you ever had a bill indicating the test is "experimental," it was due to a CMS determination. In a two-week period patients brought into my office roughly $10,000 in laboratory testing that the FDA or CMS deems "experimental" or "non-approved."

Then your doctor needs to know what they are testing for. There are definitions of false positives. You were tested and told you were positive but you were not.

And there are false negatives. Those who are indeed positive but were given a negative result. Your doctor needs to know the percentages of these tests to provide accurate results. Often, such as in the case of Lyme disease or parasites, multiple tests need to be performed due to the high amount of false negatives. There are also two other variables; specificity and sensitivity. Specificity is defined as being able to find what you're seeking. Sensitivity is defined as the percentage of actual positives one has for a test.

References ranges for any lab are calculated by standard deviation. If you have ever seen a Bell curve, ninety-seven percent falls within the curve. On the outside, three percent is outside three standard deviations.[64] [65]

One and a half percent will be a high test, and one and a half percent will be a low test. So, if you have "H's" and "L's" on your labs and your doctor says everything is fine. That's silly to me. When 98.5% of the population has a different test, there's a high percentage you're not "fine."

You may have heard of homeostasis. This is a term for how your body is supposed to function. It is a reference for what most physiology and pathology labs reference. Homeostasis is 1 standard deviation. Then, on the alternative side, there are functional ranges. These are usually calculated from two standard deviations. Outside of these ranges, but not three, you're medically fine. But this is where "pre" whatever is. I prefer to use both because I can see changes rather quick in our assessments.

There are three test choices used to evaluate hormone levels. Blood and saliva tests provide details to understand bound and unbound hormones. A urine test, known as a Dutch test, is more comprehensive and affordable. Sometimes you need to combine them for best information.

For heavy metals, a hair test only shows exposure; it doesn't show anything else, is not diagnostic, nor can you be treated from the results. Like hormone testing, there's a series of tests to see if heavy metals are an issue.

Food sensitivity panels come in many forms. There are five different antibodies, and generally, three are tested. Many national labs only test for anaphylactic IgE antibodies. Food sensitivity reports should have IgA and IgG for foods, and the individual foods need to be both raw and cooked for proper testing. This testing method is considered to be the "gold standard."

When you're paying money for these tests, you want the best testing and reporting for your money. There are quite a few doctors diagnosing parasites via dark field microscopy, heavy metals, and other tests with zero FDA or CMS approval, sensitivity, or specificity for parasitic diagnostics or other reasons. It's not even the best guess! [66] [67] [68]These are my personal observations and explanations over the past two weeks, and I'm a small clinic. Can you imagine the amount of money wasted on tests that do not provide a path to a better quality of life and don't provide valuable information for your treatment plan? You deserve the "gold standard" in laboratory testing. That is the only option we choose for our patients.

I will make a suggestion that when a test is non-routine that you ask some questions. Is it FDA approved? If insurance doesn't cover it after question one, what is the reason? How sensitive or specific is the test? Is it a gold standard?

CHAPTER 5

Your Brain is Awfully Important to Ignore

I want you to be healthy for several reasons. First, in the event you are burdened with an ill loved one or yourself to where you have to pay thousands out of pocket for the maintenance and survival, how can you do this if you are not blessed with finances? If you spend all your life's wealth accumulation in your final years, then what is left for your relatives, a charity, or whatever else your earnings could go toward to do good?

Imagine if a doctor was proactive and did their best to maintain your brain and put off dementia and Alzheimer's for a decade or more. What would that leave for your spouse, family or charity?

If you have Alzheimer's, your predicted cost per year is around $150,000. If you and your spouse have it, now it's $300,000 per year.[69] So, get out your checkbook, you're going to spend a lot. It's nearly four times as costly then if you had a stroke or other illness. Many of these costs, even now, are not reimbursed, and monthly costs are around $8,000 for family members with loved ones with

Alzheimer's and dementia versus $2,500 for those with other illnesses.

That's today's cost, what will it be in 2025? Keep in mind the foods provided in these institutions and the water. Are we stopping or promoting the process? What if I can delay these for you for a few years, how much could you pass on to your children? It's why I do what I do.

It gets a little more severe. In 2010, it was published that we are now living an average age of 78. The statistics show that once we hit 65, the chances of dementia double every five years. And once we get to 80 years old, the probability is around 50%.

WHAT TO DO: 3 Steps for Prevention

How can you prevent or reduce Alzheimer's and dementia? What can you do for yourself immediately? To prevent or reduce your Alzheimer's, one needs to understand the causes. We are now living longer than before. But the U.S. still ranks very low in longevity when compared to the other top industrialized countries. Not only are we living longer, we are living with chronic disability and inflammatory issues longer. This is due in part to better medications and health strategies.

Many of these chronic diseases you know. Alzheimer's, kidney disease, liver disease, cancers, musculoskeletal, and mental disorders to name a few. Because of new information and medical advances, those who in the past would have succumbed to their condition can now live for years with disability and some stability. But there's a cost. Individuals in this group now account for close to half of the U.S. health burden. This includes doctors visits, medications, supplements, and emergency room visits. So, we are number one in spending. Yet, the improvements in our health have not matched other wealthy nations. [70 71 72 73 74 75 76 77 78 79 80]

While I do not want you to be in this situation, there are those who unfortunately live this way every day. I feel for them. So, while I do my best to manage those cases, my goal is to prevent you, me, and anyone I know from being in this lifestyle. Going further with Alzheimer's, I've been repeating myself a lot in the office. There are several conditions that allow this to happen. First, there needs to be inflammation in the body as this is a cause for too many conditions to fester and grow. Second, exposure to copper and aluminum can make their way to the brain and take hold. Third, not having proper levels or managing blood sugar, (type III diabetes). A major cause is drinking too much fructose, mainly in the form of high fructose corn syrup.

So, to prevent Alzheimer's, you need to make sure the inflammation in your body is managed. "What do I do to manage, what is my dose?" The answer from me is, "I don't know." I have no clue about what dose you need to keep you anti-inflammatory. There are symptoms, a history that gives ideas of inflammation. But everyone is different. Any doctor who says they know are bluffing to your face. They're guessing. That is why we must run tests.[81]

That said, I do know the team players and markers in your blood tests for inflammation. We can manage what you need to have to give you the best outcome as outlined in the current research. We retest moving forward to see if those strategies are managing your physiology.

Second, you need to get yourself a filter for your water as most pipes have copper. Close to 100% of tap water has aluminum from the fluoride-treated water. Most quality filters reduce this, and of course, reverse osmosis does this better. Reverse osmosis unfortunately decreases the mineral count. So, you may need to supplement minerals if you only drink reverse osmosis water. [82] [83] [84] [85] [86] [87]

99

You want to reduce copper and aluminum as they create free radicals and target specific receptor proteins in your brain. So, you Moscow Mule enthusiasts and those cooking in copper pans, stop it! This causes brain inflammation known as neuroinflammation. Long-term neuroinflammation leads to neurodegeneration, known as Alzheimer's, dementia and Parkinson's.

Avoid monosodium glutamate (MSG) & Aspartame. "In many neurologic disorders, injury to neurons may be caused at least in part by overstimulation of receptors, from mainly glutamate and aspartate."[88] [89]

MSG, causes brain lesions in young laboratory animals and causes endocrine disturbances like obesity and reproductive disorders later in life. Sixty-six percent were more likely to have dementia, and 57% more likely to have Alzheimer's. [90]

Avoid NSAIDs if you can, or at least see if you can supplement with essential fatty acids, glutathione, and turmeric. By taking one NSAID more than every other day, users showed increased incidence of dementia and Alzheimers by 66%. [91] Risk of dementia and Alzheimer's with prior exposure to NSAIDs increases in the elderly with NSAID use.[92]

Early signs of Dementia or	Alzheimer's
Memory loss disrupting life	Forgets learned information. Forgetting important dates and events
Challenges in planning or problem solving	Errors with bank account balancing, Errors in recipes
Difficulty completing familiar tasks at home or at work	Needs help with electronics
Confusion with time or places	Loss of dates, or showing up very early or very late
Trouble understanding visual images and spatial recall	Trouble reading, judging distances
New problems with words or speaking/writing	Can't find the right word. Stops in mid-conversation
Misplacing things. Can't retrace steps	Keys, remote control, purse, where did I park?
Decreased or poor judgement	Bad grooming. Gives $ online and marketing phone scammers
Withdrawal from work or social activities	
Changes in mood and personality	

Last, you need to avoid high fructose corn syrup (HFCS). If you haven't read my articles about fructose, I encourage you to do so. In medical literature, again Alzheimer's is also known as Type III diabetes, and there is a HFCS connection. But, if you're diabetic or pre-diabetic that doesn't help either. You will want to do your best to manage and reduce your negative effects of diabetes and how it affects your brain.[93] [94]

I bring this up because unregulated diabetes wrecks your body. I'm sure you're aware of lost limbs, eyesight, and kidney loss. But, the number one cause of death to a diabetic is cardiovascular. A heart attack or stroke. The increased blood sugar scratches the arteries. Diabetes doesn't care where the arteries are, it scratches them all. So, you have a lot of arteries in your brain. Guess what? You have vessel disease here. There's a condition called vascular dementia. This is where you have many of the symptoms of Alzheimer's or another dementia, yet the cause is a lack of blood supply to those areas.

Blood supply is critical to brain function, and your brain is mostly cholesterol. I need to bring you up to speed on cholesterol, heart disease, and brain function.

Going forward, we often do more clinical tests in our office for neurological function regardless of condition. At times, you need to see a specialist while you are also helping the nutritional and physical portion of brain integrity. Yes, our office actually has a plan in place to help prevent these conditions. If you have such a condition, we do our best to maintain and manage what you have left using therapies to reconnect and grow areas in trouble. If you don't have a doctor who does this, who can test you often for any subtle changes, going once a year to a doctor for tests doesn't provide them much time or the ability to get ahead of chronic conditions. Keep in mind you will still need a filter on your water and avoid eating HCFS.

Let's get into brain specific needs. Your brain needs food! Most popular diets fail because the hypothalamus, a regulating gland in your brain, receives the starvation message. Then that starvation message signals the body to slow down metabolism. Instead, you store fat to protect against starvation and ultimately hold onto fat. What that means long term is that you have to work harder, eat less, and work out more to get this process going again. Talk about difficult. Talk about a non-functioning brain.

Your brain needs oxygen, glucose, stimulation, and a decrease in inflammation and trauma to function best. When you store fat, you aren't efficient and burning fuel and instead crave sugar to keep your engine stoked. How do you know if a program is working? How can you monitor?

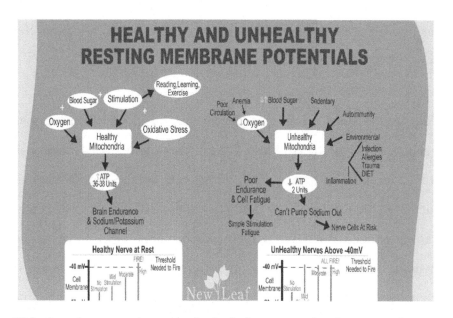

HEALTHY AND UNHEALTHY RESTING MEMBRANE POTENTIALS

This is where routine urinalysis helps one who is attempting to reduce inflammation. When you do it this way, there is a side effect of weight loss via inflammatory fat. Of course, attempting to lose weight while in a state of stress activates the adrenal gland to be in fight or flight and release cortisol and DHEA-stress hormones. When cortisol is elevated, you don't sleep. You have depression and anxiety, you decrease digestion and get gas, bloating irritable bowel, and food allergies. The immune system is suppressed and you get yeast overgrowth, allergies, and infections. You have systemic inflammation; your pancreas increases insulin and you create less energy. Then your cholesterol increases and oxidizes. This is a bad thing for cardiovascular health. And to top things off, you begin making fat around your abdomen and hips. Yay for stress! This is why weight loss is so hard. It's multi-factorial and needs a great coach who monitors urine and blood to see what you need. [95] [96]

All the previous symptoms noted are physiological processes acidifying the body. Additional symptoms of increased acidity is joint pain, mineral loss, muscle cramps and fatigue, less relaxation, increased fluid retention and fibromyalgia. You won't lose weight safely or keep it off when these are not addressed. Moreso, the hypothalamus is part of the reptilian limbic system of the brain. It contains hunger and satiny areas and is linked to both the nervous and endocrine systems by the pituitary gland. You must satisfy food, temperature, sleep, exercise, and sex to keep the hypothalamus happy. If not, you get more inflammation, brain fog, fatigue, and that foraging reflex. You know, when you're not really hungry but standing in the kitchen or pantry with the door open, wandering what to eat. That's your brain playing tricks on you.

In women, estrogen is deposited in their inflammatory yellow fat, located in their triceps, hips and thighs. Anti-inflammatory programs or nutritional changes aggressively break down yellow fat. And this stored estrogen is released back into the system. This is how a woman who was in menopause can cycle once they are in a yellow fat burning program. On the other hand, estrogen dominance occurs from too much estrogen or not enough progesterone.

Symptoms are fat stores in the tummy, hips and triceps. In men, it is in the abdomen and neck regarding excess estrogen.[97] [98]

Then what gets even more fun is you have leptin resistance on top of it. Most obese individuals have elevated levels of leptin, and the body is resisting the ability to have fat metabolism. These individuals have a decreased desire for food, increased energy expenditure, increased insulin sensitivity. While they eat less and work out more, they actually gain weight. That sucks! Leptin resistance also causes a lot of inflammation. If you're leptin resistant, you need help. I suggest a product on Full Script or something similar, EndoTrim. That will help to desensitize you to it. You will find that in our reference section. [99]

I want you to understand that it's not about cholesterol, it's about the inflammation within that cholesterol. When you have high insulin or high glucose, which is blood sugar, or high ferritin or C reactive protein, all are markers for inflammation. Any opportunity for inflammation can oxidize cholesterol in any part of your body. So, if you have inflamed joints, then you have a higher risk to oxidize your cholesterol. Thus, you have a higher risk for brain issues. Because many diseases are inflammatory such as autoimmune. Most people who are autoimmune have symptoms of brain dysfunction.[100]

When oxidation gets into your brain and causes damage, the initial term is neuroinflammation. There are two pathways to neuroinflammation. First, under an insult of inflammation, the brain by way of the immune and protective microglial cells start destruction to keep things from getting worse. It's like fighting a fire for the microglial cells. They destroy a line of trees to create a fire line so inflammation doesn't spread. Then, the second pathway that is anti-inflammatory can turn on the first pathway off and healing can begin.

But when there is chronic inflammation, it leaves the pathway for inflammation unregulated. Hence, your brain continues to be unregulated and leads to neurodegeneration. As you can see this happens overtime. This is why I want you to understand what we have in our society substances and conditions that enhance inflammation. These keep you and your family sick, whether that is sugar, trans fats, heavy metals, mold, overtraining, or overworking. They all contribute to inflammation. When you get inflammation you get oxidative stress and vice versa. This is why chronic patients in the United States are not getting the results with most doctors. They are not treating the entire person who has multiple factors affecting their health. You deserve better.

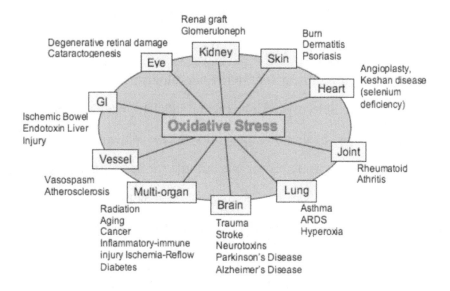

When it comes to brain health, this is something that is not working on our society. How is it that over 26% of adults in America are suffering from a mental disorder that has been diagnosed? Did you know in the last decade, the depression rates in prison rose 18%, or that total related deaths have increased by 123%? The Alzheimer's association has estimated that close to 14,000,000 Americans will have this disease in a few decades. Anxiety and depression are on the rise for all ages. They are triggers for Alzheimer's. Why? Because they are symptoms of neuroinflammation and neurodegeneration!

Published research is finding strong correlations to metals that are attacking the nervous system. They're finding them in the brains of patients who suffer from long-term neurological diseases such as ALS, Muscular Sclerosis, Alzheimer's, and Parkinson's. I have to explain that most of us are exposed to metals. When a practitioner suggests running a urine test or hair sample for heavy metals, this is not adequate. What we are looking for is that these metals have attached to a protein and the body has made an antibody.[101] [102]

There are only a few labs that run this, and what this means is that your body has created an immune response to these metals. This is bad. It's very hard to not be exposed to metals in our world. But that's what most hair and urine samples provide results for: exposure. Now what? You don't have any clue on how it affects you, if at all. This is because you don't always have to have an immune response. Instead, you can have a toxic load and need help with detoxification.

Please don't rely on hair or urine challenges for heavy metals. Unless, somehow, they are testing for antibodies and using the hair and urine for exposure findings. When you have an antibody, these immune responses create a neurotoxin which disrupts the nervous system. Now you have increased inflammation in the brain, which elicits oxidation, and in turn ages you fast and damages your DNA.

You don't get that with exposure, unless it is something very toxic, like radiation.

Which brings me up to these things called electromagnetic frequencies, or EMF. They come from your phone, laptop, tablet, Wi-Fi, microwave, and other electronic devices around us. It's estimated that one to five percent of the population already has an electromagnetic sensitivity. Also, it appears that under the influence of 5G, that the level of EMF can make you sick.[103]

Let me explain the difference in 5G compared to 4G. And now for some background on 5G. Scientists sought to test how 5G radiation is absorbed by the skin. The team, which included physicists and physicians, reached an unexpected conclusion. Using optical coherence tomography, the researchers found that sweat ducts in human skin acted as "antennas." The ducts acted as receptors for 5G radiation. Keep in mind the microwaves of cell phones are a form of radiation. Those sweat ducts, through this receptor evolution, not only capture the radiation, but concentrate and amplify it. Yuck.

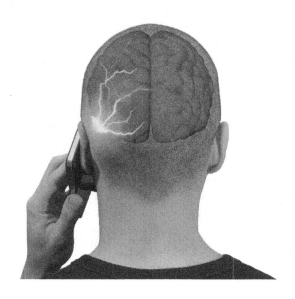

Here's where it gets more alarming. If you recall, the majority of your brain is part of the immune system containing astrocytes and glial cells which is called the microglia. Only about 10% is neurons or nerve cells. When someone has inflammation and if it's over three days, it's chronic. Most of the popular diseases that we are aware of are chronic inflammatory diseases. Alzheimer's, Parkinson's, diabetes and arthritis. So, the most important things to do is to reduce inflammation.

EMF toxicity can ramp up the glial cells and affect brain function. This means inflammation! That is the real issue with current lawsuits against cell phone companies and their 5G towers.

Microglia are nerve cells to neurons. They take care of nerve cells by protecting them and nourishing them. When they get a threat message, they ramp up fast with inflammatory cytokines much like a mama bear saving her cubs. In the act, they actually damage the nerve cells. If this can't be turned off, neuroinflammation or worse neurodegeneration of your brain is accelerated.

Microglia respond to inflammation, trauma, infections, and other assaults to the brain. At times, they induce openings in the brain in the event the brain is swelling. If you have leaky gut or leaky lung, you could have an increased lipopolysaccharide (LPS) that creates systemic inflammation and eventually glial activation. Those two pathways for glial activation from before are known as M1 and M2. One pathway is inflammatory to protect the brain and the other is for cleanup and repair. It's much the same as TH1 and TH2 in the immune system that you will get detail on later. When you have a significant amount of inflammation, or constant trauma such as in high velocity impact sports, the inflammatory protection pathway is always activated. Over time, it begins to destroy parts of the brain. Allow this to occur for several years and you have the beginning of brain degeneration. If from trauma, it's called chronic traumatic encephalopathy (CTE), as in what professional football players have. If inflammation or exposure to certain chemicals continues, your Parkinson's or Alzheimer's risk goes up. There are other causes of neurodegeneration, but these are the big ones. Most people understand because we've seen someone afflicted with them.[104] [105]

	Signs of	Parkinson's
Early	Loss of smell	Constipation
	Slow movement	Depression
	Anxiety	Stumbling
	Fatigue	Sleep issues
Progressed signs	Decreased dexterity	Writing cramps
	Soft Voice	Slurring words
Disease state	Resting tremor	Dementia
	Expressionless face	Rigidity

A lot of people can't feel what is affecting them or their brain. Otherwise we wouldn't smoke, drink, consume HFCS, junk food, or do silly things that destroy our bodies. EMF is no different. The U.S. National Toxicology Program started a study in 2016 that looked at ten years of cell phone use. They published their consensus that cell phones have carcinogenic effects. The International Agency for Research on Cancer found normal cell phone use increased gliomas by 40% over time. If you remember, those glial cells—immune protectors of the brain—are now attacking the brain. While there are many cancers, this is dangerous and malignant 80% of the time. [106]

With your cell phone, there are three types of wireless functions. Cellular (the G's), Bluetooth, and Wi-Fi. For most phones, Airplane Mode disables them all. But newer phones you have to disable them one at a time. Keep in mind there is strength in the proximity of your phone. So, holding it directly to your face or ear is the worse possible option. Speakerphone gives you the most distance should you need to use your phone.

A missing signal bar could be an issue. It is recommended to use your phone outside or near a window. In the basement or area of low signal, some phones ramp up emission by up to 1,000 times to grab a signal. This could be increased exposure for one individual compared to another.

Let's get into brain-based nutrition needs. Brain-specific nutrition is more than just taking something that has been researched for the brain. It's a lot more complicated and multi-factorial than this. Also, this goes for most conditions. If you get an ad that says take this one thing to relieve this, and it comes with a myriad of testimonials, do you research. Have their claims been published? What about with certain conditions? Do they interact with medications?

Before I get into specific nutrition, the best thing for your brain is sleep. You will see this again later, so hold on to it. If you sleep next to an LED light, such as in an alarm clock, or a light in the room, this affects your melatonin and good sleep. You want a dark room. Black out shades are not a requirement, but a great recommendation. Also, keep those devices away from you. If you must have a phone for an alarm or emergency call, leave it in the room but as far away as possible in night mode or airplane mode.

If you have a diet where you eat lead or aluminum or work in an industry that has them. Be aware, these metals can interfere with brain function. You can get lead from lead pipes, batteries, soil, dust, foreign candy, bullets, weights, and paint. Also, lead can interfere with brain-derived neurotrophic factors, how you brain heals. This is one of the reasons lead was removed from paint several decades ago. Aluminum comes in cans, dental devices, wrappers, foil, and other food sources. You can increase BDNF with high intensity exercise, sleep, and stress reduction. If you have mold, gas leaks, or other toxins in the house, you can't supplement your way to health. If they're suspected, get your home tested so you can make the best decision on where to spend your money for your health. [107] [108]

There is a lot of connection for your health and brain to your teeth. The nerves to your teeth fire directly into your brain and have a connection to the organ systems. The health of the mouth affects the vagus nerve, which is a control center of your autonomic nervous system and regulates elimination, digestion, and reproduction, to name a few.

Because your brain is mostly fat, you want non-inflammatory good fats in your diet. This could be medium chain triglycerides (MCT), organic virgin coconut oil, avocado oil, and extra virgin olive oil. There are few others that make the list, so if you don't know if it's a good fat, it probably isn't. Some people choose fish oil as their main fat. That's a great idea. Here are some fun facts to know when choosing a fish oil.

Where is it from? Organic or not?

Is the oil exposed or tested for mercury, as many large cold-water fish have mercury? Is the oil stabilized with an anti-oxidant vitamin E blend known as mixed-d-alpha tocopherols? If not, that mega bottle of fish oil with exposure to air, once oxidized, becomes rancid. So, about one third of the bottle is actually worthless, if not harmful. This is how one study can say fish oil or vitamin E is great for the heart and another says it's dangerous. It's all about the stability and if they are oxidized or not. We do not want oxidation.

Is it EPA or DHA or both? For inflammation, we want more EPA. For the brain, we want more DHA. Sometimes we want both or a blend. For patients with massive inflammation I start with EPA. [109 110]

For kids and patients with brain fog and no real inflammatory markers in their blood, I generally advise more DHA. Don't get me wrong, you need both. [111 112 113 114]

Then there are the antioxidants. Remember, there is not a blood test for this. But you have inflammation markers that do respond to anti-oxidants. So, you take what you can afford until the markers and symptoms improve. This group consists of alpha lipoic acid, turmeric, resveratrol, coQ-10, ubiquinol, hepcidin, and vinpocetine. There are others like Vitamin C, but these are the heavy hitters. Many of these can support blood supply and get it to the brain more efficiently. [115]

Some people and doctors chose B vitamins as their method of choice. Or, when we get into genetics, individuals find they have an MTHFR gene mutation. They slam back B12 or Folate with recklessness. I'll explain more in genetics, but you are defined by more than one gene. B vitamins are good for the methylation and rebuilding your cycle. There is a time and place for them for brain and cardiovascular health.

At times, hormones need to be balanced for the brain. But, and this is a big one, inflammation is the main cause of imbalanced hormones. So, throwing more hormones into the mix doesn't get the job done. More than not, it's the equivalent of throwing gasoline on a fire.

Brain Testing

The "E" eye chart almost everyone is familiar with was developed in 1862. It's called the Snellen chart after its inventor, the Dutch ophthalmologist Herman Snellen. While today most doctors use the updated LogMAR chart, it does the same thing: measures how well we see static images at a distance of 20 feet. Yet, because we rely on vision while our eyes, bodies, or objects are in motion. Only about five percent of vision problems are found with an eye chart! This testing method is insufficient for everyone—children, in particular. I haven't found a child with ADD or ADHD that doesn't have trouble with their vision. Sometimes it's as easy as changing the diet. For others, it's blue-light blocking glasses, and some need supplements. Rarely, and I reiterate rarely, do they need medications to increase focus and communication? Because the eyes are a window into the brain, it's a good place to start, but not finish.

So what's the deal with neurofeedback? Neurofeedback takes advantage of the fact that the brain can change. It can be plastic, meaning that you can retrain it to be more efficient, or in some cases, less responsive. Neurofeedback can help dampen the response of the amygdala (part of the reptilian brain.) It will be less responsive and less dominant. With the amygdala out of the way, the better we deal with adversity. We are more efficient persons when we allow our prefrontal cortex to deal with emotions. These are empathy, compassion, and more important, executive decisions. This is how somebody can feel paralyzed when they have a bunch of stuff thrown at him at once and they literally do not know what to do. A good Neurofeedback (NF) device runs about $20,000, and that's not reasonable for most people. Neither is a standard laser that encompasses neurofeedback and brain waves. The most affordable one that I can find still runs the $6,500.[116]

There are some brain-specific home devices that work well and in our appendix. Because neurofeedback puts your brain in a place it does not want to be, you may not want to jump right in. It's more helpful for starters to do an activity that you can't do or struggle

119

with. That could be playing the piano. You could learn a language, or tell your ex you forgive them. That way you're exercising at home and managing your amygdala, thus, making it efficient.

Besides, NF meditation appears to be one of the best methods to calm your amygdala. Twenty minutes today doesn't sound like much. Unless you're monitoring how you sleep and how you respond to stress, you may consider meditation. You can monitor that with the HRV device while you're doing mindful meditation and breathing exercises at the same time. You can still get stressed out about certain things, but it doesn't have to be internal. What meditation does neurologically is to help support the hippocampus. This is most of your short-term memory. But there are other parts of the hippocampus, such as the left side, that can help with long-term and flexibility in your thinking.

Regular, consistent exercise and an anti-inflammatory diet are essential to increase each persons' longevity and brain function. For exercise, use high intensity from our reference chart. It doesn't take much. Sometimes as little as 3-5 minutes a day.

Our food sources are where you could be getting exposed to these toxins, and it can get you into trouble. Many of these foods have their genetics modified for more growth and yield (GMO). The top crops that are GMO and have infiltrated our food supply are soy, corn, and beats. Also, in oils such as cottonseed and canola, which are in many of the processed foods. When you're shopping, look for organic food. I get it, sometimes you can't find it. Other times it's a budget issue. I ask you to keep in mind eating more organic as opposed to more GMO will reduce toxic chronic inflammation. This will save you money in the long run. You will miss less work or being sick less eating non-GMO inflammatory foods. Many of your GMO's have been exposed to a chemical called glyphosate. Is very hard to stay away from that stuff and one of the main reasons we use liposomal glutathione in our office. Glyphosate is the active ingredient in Roundup. You may have heard of it before. It's even modified as part of the seed to prevent pets and other growth deterrents. The problem is that we can't get away from it. We can't wash it off. It's in our food and it's DNA. In a nutshell, glyphosate is a massive free radical.[117] [118]

CBD

Let's take a moment to talk about CBD. The main question is how you can get high on it? You can't. It doesn't have THC that is the part of the cannabis plant that gets you high. Hemp doesn't contain it and you can't get high. You need 100 mg of THC or more that gets a psychotropic effect. How CBD works is by actions on different parts of the brain through what's called neurotransmitters. These influence that ECS system, otherwise known as Endocannabinoids. You have an ECS system through your entire body as a regulator, modulator, and connector through your hormones and immune system. CBD acts on two main receptors known as CVD1 and CBD2. With CVD1 found in the brain, and the organs have CBD2. CBD is known to aid serotonin which is a natural antidepressant, appetite suppressant, and mood regulator. Serotonin works become melatonin for better sleep. For those who have ADD, they are low on their ECS system, which means they have low dopamine. In neurotransmitters, CBD enhances dopamine and helps focus and concentration.[119]

The big deal with ECS is that it has a role in inflammation, sleep, anxiety, and energy. New research is showing this connection to the brain, and in turn, helping the digestion by tightening up junctions in the intestines. It's a permeable membrane, or in layman's terms, a leaky gut aide. It won't fix a gut forever, but it can have a positive effect. Assuming you have been taking an NSAID that has been destroying your gut, CBD may be a viable option for you.

I can't tell you how skeptical I was at first with CBD. It fixed everything? Nonsense. Well, it doesn't. It helps the brain with inflammation. Isn't that anxiety and depression? Isn't that how the nervous system gets its information? The information for pumping blood, digestion, immunity, pain blocking?

It's not an end all, and you will likely need other supplements and therapies with it, but I can't deny the research. CBD is to come with no psychotropic effects nor the marijuana substance to cause that THC. Is your company testing for that? An FYI, testing for THC for many companies is considered zero at 99.7% so there could be a minute amount of THC. So, if you have a THC sensitivity that could be a problem. But it's not close to the 100 mg or more to get a psychotropic effect.[120]

When it comes to absorption, should you take a tincture, should it be mixed with MCT oil for the brain in a gummy form, paste, lotion, or a capsule. It's actually how you will take it. If you don't like the taste, you may not continue. That said, it's fat soluble. So, I prefer my recommended delivery systems to be in a fat such as MCT or coconut oil for internal issues. Or as a lotion for topical pain.

CBD dosing doesn't depend on body size or weight, male, or female. Some people need a lot, and some need very little. It's all about the function of your ECS. Our government has issued the use of CBD as an antioxidant. I know I didn't put it in the section above because it's a Jack of all Trades acting as more than an antioxidant.

Not all CBD is created equal. While CBD is a master regulator and can affect many systems of the body, not knowing what CBD to take could be a problem. CBD can be used across the spectrum from children to adults. It's not a cure for everything by a long stretch, but it can help regulate issues, especially the ECS system in the body. When choosing a CBD company, find one that will provide you with clinical specs. Trust me when I say this, very few have them. I'm asking for pesticides, arsenic, heavy metals, toxins, mold, and other impurities that I do not want in my body. The company we prefer is in our reference section, but you can use the above questions to keep you safe. Each company should have specs testing for their products, and they keep it clean from their suppliers to you.

Advanced Vision/Brain Testing

Many people have memory issues, brain fog, lack of focus, or have trouble reading. If you suffer from headaches, brain fog, problems with coordination, or a feeling of "off" or "just not right", these are examples of how a person's health is affected by vision problems.

In our office, we use a device called RightEye because it picks up subclinical brain dysfunction by tracking eye movements. Sometimes your symptoms are metabolic, such as blood supply to the brain, anemia, or lack of exercise. These all lead to not getting enough oxygen into your lungs, and at times, the nervous system hasn't been exercised.

Vision is more than 20/20 eyesight as stated before. Our visual abilities impact every aspect of our lives. Our balance, hand-eye coordination, reading comprehension, and reaction time can be compromised when our vision is impaired. A brain function can deteriorate even the smallest impairment. Hand-eye coordination tasks requiring acute visual focus include hitting a golf ball, driving, catching a baseball, sewing, and chopping vegetables to name a few. Why? Vision and visual acuity are not the same as your eyesight. A person with 20/20 vision may still show signs of weak eye movement and eye tremor behaviors.

RightEye is an eye-tracking system for general health and wellness. It is fast and accurate to assess functional vision and brain health in ways that are impossible with the standard Snellen eye test. The test is painless. It only takes a few minutes and provides a wealth of information.

RightEye software uses advanced eye-tracking technology to identify a wide variety of vision issues impacting your quality of life. You can link the efficiency of your eye movement to your brain health. Eye-tracking technology, which is objective and non-invasive, captures high-speed pictures of eye movements (30-250) times each second. You could have perfect vision. Yet, you might have brain fog or brain fatigue with other activities such as exercise or reading. That's so frustrating to my patients. Especially when they've been multiple places, and no one has picked up on this yet.

RightEye testing works by linking eye movement and eye function to brain performance. Involuntary eye movements are often not apparent to the naked eye. So, we miss these as doctors during your eye exam. But they are a clear indication of both visual performance and many other health issues. By measuring and analyzing these hidden patterns, doctors using RightEye and similar devices can identify dysfunctions. This is important for you. One has to find what is not working to treat you. Once they know what isn't working, they should offer treatment options to correct a wide array of vision and health issues, not to mention improve global visual performance.

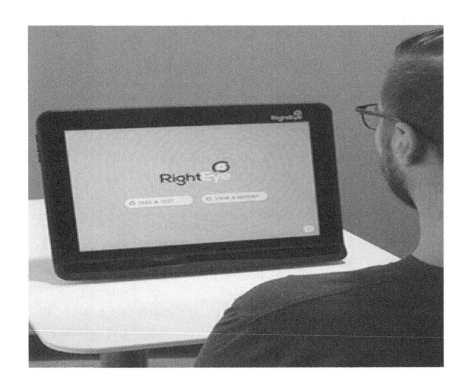

The data produced in the RightEye test is quantitative—meaning it allows physicians to identify vision and health issues in a measurable way. We get to know when you're better and when you can do more. This is huge for people with learning disorders, dyslexia, ADD, ADHD, depression, anxiety, brain fog, fatigue, balance, brain injuries, and memory issues. This technology can assess and improve the experiences of athletes, track recovery and identify improvements before they get hurt or allowed to participate too early[121 122 123 124 125].

So, when we find these things in our office, or a patient comes in stating they have them and want help, we have to find out why, often I start with development. Sure, this is much easier in a one-year-old or even a five-year-old, but your development is vital to what part of the brain developed best and what could use some help. Below is a chart on milestones in development. When a child talks, walks, or feeds themselves late, they have a developmental delay in that area. I understand we "grow" out of it. Shoot, I didn't talk until I was four and didn't walk until two. Our doctor said I was lazy and would figure it out. Well, it happened. I walked and talked. But here's the bigger picture. Those areas of my brain did not develop at the same rate as my peers. Luckily, my mother was a big proponent of reading and music. And my father worked a lot with hand eye coordination, even though I always felt he threw a ball too hard. They were working on my left-brain and right-brain interconnectivity, but didn't know they were.

Child	Development			
0-1 year	Sip from cup	Sit alone	Babble	Smile
	Peek-a-boo	Roll over	Pulls up	Understand "No"
1-3 years	Feeds self	Walk, run, pivor	Say name	Name pictures
	Dresses self	Imitates others	Uses spoon	Echoes words
	Recognizes colors	Uses more words	Male female	differences
3-6 years	Draw circle square	Skip	Stick figure drawing	Balance-bicycle
	Catch a ball	Independent	Hops on 1 foot	Gets time concept
6-12 years	Team sports	Menarche	Peer recognition	Reading skills
	Has a routine	Knows directions	Loses baby teeth	
12-18 years	Adult looking	Acne	Peer acceptance	Comprehension

There is one caveat in development I get from a lot of parents, so I feel it's important to put in here. Often, a parent is in the office with their child or talking about a sibling and stating, "Last week they just reverted back to XYZ." While this is alarming, hold onto that thought. If there wasn't a major trauma, medication change or illness there is another reason, I'm sure if you ask your parents, you did the same thing. Sometimes it's bedwetting, or a stutter, or spilling water for an entire week and then it went away. There is some science behind this. It's called brain pruning. When you develop a brain, it branches out for new connections and neuroplasticity. Think of the growing brain of a child like a shrub. At times the apical bud or some of the branches take off and grow much faster than the rest. Your brain comes along and "prunes" off the lengthened branches. The result, there is a day to a week of regression. This is normal. However, longer than that you need to see someone, or in the case of an accident, go see someone.[126]

Fast forward 40 years later. When I've been working too long or pushing myself, I revert back to my three-year-old self. I become isolated, not wanting to nap or take a break, grumpy and irritable. I don't talk. Please don't ask me questions and no, I do not want to be told what to do!

I'm sure we all have these issues to some degree with fatigue. During my insane exercise days of marathons, ultramarathons and triathlons, I was a three-year-old. I was torching my brain with excess free radicals and I couldn't make or take enough antioxidants to keep up. I was a mess. Don't get me wrong. If it is on your bucket list to do one of these events, have at it. Keep in mind there is no healthy way to do a marathon or other endurance sport. [127]

Your brain has several parts. I won't get into all the connections and specific locations, but an overview is warranted to help you understand what may or may not be working. The majority of your brain is called the cortex. There is a left and right hemisphere, left brain right brain, and at the bottom, a cerebellum with cranial nerves coming from a brain stem.

The cortex has different areas. The front is called the frontal lobe. The middle is the parietal lobe. Around your ears, the temporal lobe, and at the back your occipital lobe. Each lobe has specific functions, but they all integrate and tell the cerebellum what is happening. The more plasticity you have, the better the function. The less inflammation and trauma to your glial cells and astrocytes, the better the function.

Parts of the Human Brain

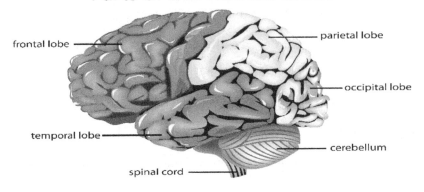

If you have trouble in your frontal lobe, you will have issues with determination, perception, appreciation, motor control, and motivation. Also, problem solving, language skills, and impulse control. This is where ADD and ADHD reside the most. Yes, they can have chemical and metabolic imbalances, but this is the lobe that is affected for those conditions. The frontal lobe is where you have your personality, the food you like, the music you listen to. If you don't use it, you lose it. So, if you're a couch potato and you don't use any motor control, now you can see how a loss in that can exhibit symptoms of personality changes, laziness, loss in motivation, and loss of impulse control.

Your temporal lobe is where you hear. It also houses a portion called the hippocampus. This is mainly for short term memory. Combined with the frontal lobe, these areas are generally what shows up first in Alzheimer's. You also get conversion from short term to long term memory. So, if you have ringing in the ears, or your short-term memory is having an issue, perhaps you should look into helping your temporal lobe.

The parietal lobe is about midway in your brain between the frontal lobe (motor) and is the main sensory part of your brain. You also recognize faces, numbers, and shapes with this. You interpret speech, touch, vibration, temperature, and pain. Here's the problem discerning early dementia and parietal lobe issues without a thorough evaluation. If the parietal lobe is hurt from a concussion, then you are slow to recognize a ball coming at you and your friends. You are slow to send a signal to your temporal lobe. You can't recognize the potential danger, and you're slow to relay information to your frontal lobe to move or yell, "Look out."

Neurology is more than just a form or a few tests, and not everyone is wired the same way. It's a global examination looking at every possibility and finding what can make an immediate impact to help your neuroplasticity.

At the back of your head is the occipital lobe. This is where you see. The occipital lobe discriminates colors and light. It helps with depth perceptions and it coordinates with the parietal lobe on what you see. This is how a blow to the back of the head can leave someone blind.

The cerebellum is at the bottom of the brain, and this is where we see the most issues. As I get into the autoimmune section, so many Americans have issues here and don't even know they have signs of neurodegeneration. The cerebellum is responsible for balance, but more importantly, it takes all the information from the other lobes and decides what to do. You have millions of receptors from your brain and your body bombarding the cerebellum at any given time. Ninety percent of the information provided is not used. This is the part of the brain that is susceptible to alcohol and why police use it for sobriety testing, even though alcohol affects all parts. This is also where gluten and those with certain autoimmune conditions and most thyroid conditions go and attack this part of the brain.

Now you can see why you are having more and more anxiety and depression. How this can increase neurodegenerative diseases when our food, lifestyles, and exposures affect this very important part of the brain.

Below the cerebellum is your brain stem that has cranial nerves. These are responsible for smell, taste, digestion, eye movement, bite, chewing, facial expression, hearing, tongue movement, and swallowing. I bring up the parts of the brain so you can identify specific issues to talk to your doctor or go through an at-home course. We offer webinars of many of the subjects in this book, but so do other well-known doctors. I want to empower you to see the big picture and motivate you before it's too late to do anything.

Your brain also runs the autonomic nervous system (ANS). The ANS consists of two parts known as parasympathetic and sympathetic. Again, parasympathetic is defecation, reproduction, immunity, blood supply, and digestion. Sympathetic is fight or flight. It gets your heart to pump blood to lungs and major muscles. It helps you sweat when you are nervous, pump adrenalin, and keep you alive under stress and impending doom. The problem is too many people live in a sympathetic state. When you do that, the parasympathetic is turned off and sub-functional.

Regarding the ANS, your mind plays a critical role. You could balance the ANS through religious conviction and/or mental and emotional connections. Quality sleep, healthy relationships, laughing, loving, and crying all balance the ANS. Even your thoughts can inhibit or enhance your physiology. Remember the lemon story?

When it comes to brain function, how to exercise that thought process is important for you. Either through body or eye exercise, nutrition, diet and other lifestyle changes can make huge impacts on your brain. This is the difference on whether you maintain and improve or continue to degenerate at your current rate.

In conclusion, for your brain, you must make sure the metabolic rate is working. Be tested for anemia, inflammation, and blood sugar handling. Look back and see if you started down this road with exposure to something, an illness, infection, or diagnosis. Maybe you moved into a new place or new state with a different season. Take note of what you are eating. Understand that the rate is also important. Did it happen over the last 30 years or the last 30 days? Do you have a family history of neurodegeneration or bout of anxiety or depression? Do you exercise or over exercise? Can you get your normal daily tasks completed, or is this a challenge? These are great questions to decide if you need further help beyond this book. If you don't see improvement or you're getting worse, see someone ASAP!

CHAPTER 6

Your Immune System

O ne of the biggest questions I get today is what can I do for my immunity? Technically, that's a loaded question, because I don't know your case or your life history and all the variables that go into your immune system. Let's start with some education and understand how the immune system works so we know what we can focus on.

Immune Resilience

Part of your immune system is the ability to ward off pathogens and prevent you from getting an infection. The term for this is immune resilience. Simply having an illness or having an autoimmunity doesn't mean that you have lost your resilience. But you can have multiple people with the same disease living in the same home. They could work in the same area, eat the same food, and have the same lifestyle, yet all have different immune functions. Some people have elevated white blood cell counts and some people have decreased white blood cell counts. That tells us that there are different parts of their immune system working. Your immune system has several pathways such as TH1, TH2, TH3, and TH17.

It's more complicated then this explanation, but here is your immune system in a nutshell. One pathway handles manufacturing antibodies. Another is for killing the pathogen. Another to influence inflammation and another for balancing all of them.

Immune system regulation

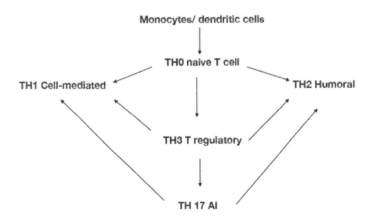

Autoimmunity

For many people today, they are trying to boost their immune systems and are reading about any product that will bolster their immune system. It's a lot more complicated, especially if your autoimmune. And for those people, there's a more in-depth topic later on specific to autoimmunity.

If you never have heard of autoimmunity or don't completely understand it, that's okay. Most people with autoimmunity don't even know they have autoimmunity.[128]

The big ones are autoimmune diseases such as diabetes, rheumatoid arthritis, psoriasis, Crohn's, and celiac. You know about it because of the multitude of commercials on TV. Actually, there are about 120 more autoimmune conditions that, when defined, mean your immune system is attacking yourself. There is a lot more to read regarding autoimmunity and it's a chapter of its own. These are the basic concepts.

The medical term is a loss of self-tolerance because your immune system no longer knows what is you and what is not you, hence the term autoimmune. Your immune system attacks you, the host. When you make more efficient killer cells, you become more efficient in response to infections. Killer cells kill invaders. That's their role. They get more efficient if antibodies "tag" their prey. But, they don't always need antibodies to go to work. Consider antibodies a laser-guided missile. They are much more precise and accurate. Natural killer cells are more like cluster-bombing in WW2. Lots of damage, but not very accurate.

There are those who have their immune system making antibodies and not killer cells. They are less efficient to respond to infections. It comes down to your killer cells. Antibodies help natural killer cells find the invader and then kill what they are attached to. But, if you make antibodies to yourself, then they do their job, they then attack you.

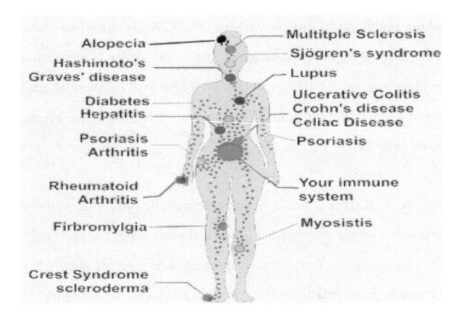

Antibodies and Pathways

Going back to the pathways above, there are supplements to support each side and pathway. If your body is making too many antibodies and you take a supplement that helps support that pathway, you will get worse and make more antibodies.

The same will happen if you have tissue destruction and you take a supplement that supports the pathway for tissue destruction. Yes, they are immune boosting supplements! Keep in mind 75% of Americans have some degree of autoimmunity. [129]

So I tend to look at the big picture and ask a lot of historical questions to get an idea what I'm dealing with in the office. That may not be workable for everyone in today's world.

Autoimmune Versus Immunocompromised

Many autoimmune patients voice concern that they don't have any resilience or are more susceptible to getting sick. Yet they haven't been sick or had a cold in years. The reality is these patients have an elevated immune system. And then there are others, who every time someone has a cold in the office, or a child they know gets sick, they get sick. Most of these individuals have low white blood counts, generally under five. That does not mean that they are immunocompromised and cannot fight off infections.

Generally speaking, the higher the white blood cell count means that they have a higher amount of natural killer cells. The individuals have a better ability to fight off infections. For them, autoimmunity has helped them, and for those who get sick all the time, autoimmunity has not helped them.

So, what is immunocompromised? When we test your blood, one of the markers is white blood cell count. Normal is 5-8. The definition of immunocompromised is when your white blood cell count is below 2.5. So, as you can see, having an autoimmune disease does not mean that you are immunocompromised. In some cases, having a pathogen is actually protective for autoimmune conditions for a short time.

We see this in a parasite when compared to the flu. There is emerging evidence that parasites help balance autoimmunity, whereas the flu can make your autoimmunity worse. Please don't go looking for one, at least not yet. If you have a low white count, you need to educate yourself about what can help your immune system.

Other than social distancing, what can help your resilience towards infections? Are there other factors that can slow down your immune system even further? The next few paragraphs are generalities for everyone. No one will react the same way, and this isn't a personalized plan for your immunity. Every pathogen has its own pathway, every individual has our own genetics. Everyone has their own lifestyle that contributes either positive or negative to their immunity and health outcomes.

Immune System Basics

Other than particular supplements, there are five subsets that are very important to keep your immune system running regardless of genetics, sex, or ethnicity. Everyone needs sleep, blood sugar handling, hydration, exercise, and stress management. At the end of this, I will also provide a link to supplements that have research showing that they benefit the immune system. This does not mean you will be immune to everything and you still need to have some common sense when dealing with the public. Consider supplements like routine maintenance on your car, or flossing your teeth. These things will break down over time. But do some self-maintenance now to extend that time and help your immune system become more efficient, period.

1 Sleep

First subset is sleep. How much and how restful your sleep is the number one factor that will help support or destroy an immune system. There are multiple causes for lack of sleep. While there are supplements out there that help sleep, they are not a long-term solution and should only be used in the intermediate, and not long term, until you figure out why you are not sleeping. If you don't have any white noise in your bedroom, that's another key factor. The sound needs to be continuous and not a rainforest, animal sounds or a thunderstorm. You also need it dark as possible with limited electronic devices on. Decrease your room temperature to below 70, and you have set the mood for sleep.

There are a few other ways to help your brain function naturally so you can get to sleep using science. If you have LED lights, they can affect your brain waves. They can also penetrate curtains.

You need dark to rest and repair. Your cells that see light are active ,and this ages you faster because they can't rest.

Our infrastructure of today changes our biological clocks. It's dark outside, but I'll turn on a light. That's disruptive to your health. Blue light, from our devices, shuts down melatonin production which is critical for falling asleep. It gets more precise. There are times during the day your genes make more proteins for hormones such as you thyroid, liver, and kidney. Exposure to artificial light or not enough sunlight affects hormone production.

Here are the main reasons for not getting enough sleep:

A. Screen time

Staying up late on devices too long. Use the f.lux app on your electronics and night, and use blue-light blocking glasses after sunset.[130]

B. Caffeine consumption

Too much caffeine consumption throughout the day or caffeine consumption too late in the evening affects sleep.[131]

C. Weak pelvic floor

There's another reason that people get up in the night and that is because they have a weak pelvic floor. When that happens, they have to get up and go to the bathroom one to 10 times in the night. Other than seeing a chiropractor to balance the pelvis, I recommend you go online and look at pelvic floor exercises. You shouldn't spend more than a few minutes on these a day. You'll want to do these for two straight weeks to see if that makes a difference. If you're one of those who gets up at night to go to the bathroom, start counting how many times you're getting up. After two weeks, see if it decreased.

You can also use these easy solutions to get your rhythm back in sync.

1. Do a 20-30 min walk outside after sunrise upon waking.

2. Reduce contacts, glasses, and sunglasses when you can and if you can. These decrease sunlight that tells your brain it's work time.

3. Open windows and allow more natural light in.

4. Use orange/red lightbulbs in the evening, or candlelight, or start the fireplace in the evening. These low light evening options set in motion sleep hormones.

5. Do relaxing therapies like neurofeedback, emotional freedom, eye movement desensitization, reprocessing, meditation, or ho'oponopono a Hawaiian emotional release..

6. If you don't have any white noise in your bedroom, that's another key factor. The sound needs to be

continuous and not a rainforest, animal sounds, or a thunderstorm.

7. Stabilize your blood sugar so you can do intermittent fasting. If you have high (hyperglycemia) or low (hypoglycemia), both affect sleep. Either high or low is called dysglycemia and is the second subset for dysfunctional immunity.

2. Blood Sugar Ups and Downs: Dysglycemia

The reality is low blood sugar/hypoglycemia is the main cause for a lack of sleep. But it, along with diabetes, also drains your immune system.[132]

Many of the above options are a pretty easy fix, but how do you fix low blood sugar? First, let's talk about some of the symptoms of low blood sugar so that you have an idea of what that looks like.

The term for low blood sugar is hypoglycemia. It comes in levels of severity from temporary and short-lived bouts, or until you eat, or throughout the day. Hypoglycemia can come with brain usage, more commonly known as thinking. Most people who are hypoglycemic feel better after they eat. Or, when they wake up, they are not hungry. They often get dizzy, shaky, or light headed between meals.

146

The first fix to that is to make sure you're eating breakfast and that your breakfast consists of protein. If that doesn't take care of it, you'll need to eat more throughout the day. That doesn't mean more calories, it means you're sitting down and eating more times. It is legal to split a meal into two different sessions of eating.

When you have hypoglycemia, you have a low adrenal response. Therefore, you have low blood supply, meaning you will have low immunity and often low blood pressure. It's a big deal for immunity. You have a lower response because you can't move the blood, containing those natural killer cells, to where they are supposed to be. If you're always cold, is that blood nourishing your brain? Probably not.[133]

Those who are hypoglycemic should never fast. There is a time and a place for an imminent fasting. But I can't see it anytime when you're hypoglycemic and/or have the symptoms above. In some cases, I have hypoglycemic patients eat before they go to bed so that they have fuel for their brain to help fall and stay asleep.

Fasting

Regarding fasting there's plenty of research that supports it improves your immune system. Why? Because it decreases oxidative stress. Do not fast if you are hypoglycemic. But if you're diabetic and test hyperglycemic, this can be wonderful for your immune system. Fasting can decrease free radicals and then your antioxidant stores go up. Antioxidants are protective to your immune system, brain, and digestion. Without a doubt, fasting protects the immune system. But not if you're hypoglycemic!

3. Dehydration

The third biggest stress on the immune system that I see in my office is dehydration. Hydration is important for the immune interactions, and how it communicates. If you're dehydrated, your lymphatic system is less efficient. Proper hydration moves the chemical messengers called cytokines through your body. Hydration allows your immune system to communicate more effectively. Dehydration decreases this communication which limits your ability to respond.

Here are some highlights for hydration and some rules to consider. If you drink water and feel better, that's a sign of dehydration. If you're thirsty, that's another sign. When you urinate, it should be clear, not dark. We get dehydrated at night, so our morning urination is often darker. Here's a good reason to start the day with a glass of water.

When you have an infection, it is important to stay hydrated and you should try to drink throughout the entire illness.

While certain coffees and tea can support the immune system, they are also diuretics, meaning that they dehydrate you. So, if you're drinking these things, you have to drink more water. Also, alcohol and salt are diuretics. A rule for drinking liquids that are also diuretics is that you must double the amount of water for what you're consuming. For instance, if you drink an 8-ounce cup of coffee, then you will have an eight ounce diuretic, so you need to drink 16 ounces of water to be eight ounces ahead. The drink in this case does not count, it only subtracts. To stay hydrated, your ideal consumption of water should be three to four liters per day, which is roughly 100-120 ounces for an adult of about 140 pounds. Make changes for different sizes of adults and children.

If you work out, which is our next topic, you will need to drink more water. Drinking sports drinks that are full of sugar or have caffeine in them can impair your immune system. There are plenty of studies that show that drinking one soda pop turns off your white blood cell production between 24 and 36 hours!

If you're not sick, you can exercise longer, but if you're fighting something, a few minutes of some movement will be sufficient. Our office provides patients with urinary strips to check for proper hydration, detoxification, infection, inflammation, and loss of sugar. Of all the tests we run, one of the easiest and informative tests is a urinalysis.

4. Exercise

So let's talk about exercise. One needs the proper blood flow for the immune system to work, and exercise can help with that. But what exercise should you be doing? How long should you be doing it? The fundamental variable is your heart rate. You want your heart rate to come up to have benefit. If your exercise raises your heart rate by slow movement, that could be ok in yoga or Pilates, because it should rise with the duration of exercise. If your movement is so slow that your heart rate hardly changes, that's not considered exercise. You need to increase blood flow. This increases the immune chemical and lymphatic circulation to improve your immune system.

When you get sick, sometimes you have lymphatic tissue that swells and is often hot or tender. That lymph node is providing your immune system information and is now waiting for instruction. Movement helps your messengers get to your lymph node and have a positive effect.

Yoga

Yoga is a great exercise for all people. If you are autoimmune, hot yoga can do two things that affect your immune system in a negative way. First, it can dehydrate you and the heat creates cortisol, your stress hormones. There are plenty of online classes, paid and free channels that are for children, beginners, and experts. Remember, a muscle needs to have strength, coordination, and flexibility. While you can get all that in yoga, you may still need to incorporate weight training for extra strength and muscle tone.

Weight Lifting

If you lift weights, that's great, but you're missing flexibility and coordination. I prefer weight that can go from low to high without taking a ton of space. You need to add some balance and mixed activities such as push-ups with the hands not level, or lift on a balance board. Not one exercise is perfect for everyone, but we all need to try other ones so that our muscles don't get memory and become inefficient. Challenge your muscles to fire in different ways, it's a big deal.

Endurance Exercise

For those who love endurance activities such as running, biking or swimming, the tendency is to go for a very long time. Please don't, unless you are getting ready for a big event or getting paid. There are so many endurance athletes that are as close to the walking dead because they overtrain, undernourished, and are dehydrated. These are all great setups for disaster for your physiology, if not autoimmunity. We often have to break things down by heart rate or duration. You should shoot on recovery days if you are very fit to keep your heart rate below 150 beats per minute, or under 130 if you've just started your exercise journey. This allows you a chance to recover. Obviously, running up hills, doing intervals, or racing ,the heart rate is going to be much higher than that. You can do these, but keep it within reason. Too much and you'll make inflammatory changes that make it harder to recover and stay healthy.

Over-Exercise

Exercise itself has positive effects on the pathways above. No matter what, you will make free radicals when you exercise, which can decrease the immune system. It's important to focus on exercise that limits free radicals and boosts a surge of antioxidants. These are the molecules that block free radicals for hours after your exercise.

The best type of exercise to support your immune system is high intensity training otherwise known as HIT. There are plenty of online websites where you can get where you can get intense, HIT training. These are not what I am talking about. You need between five and 20 minutes of HIT training a day and I've included a fantastic for this (LINK: https://8fit.com/dralantrites). This does not mean you have to give up yoga, Pilates, running, cycling or anything else that you love to do for exercise. What it means is if you exercise too hard or too long, you have a negative effect on your immune system and that's not the point in today's world. This is not High Intensity Interval Training. HIIT is a lot more intense. Programs like "insanity" or crossfit. I don't support those for health and immunity. I have treated too many injuries, and from years of blood tests, and office visits there's not enough benefit. Sure, you may look good, but you're not healthy.[134] [135]

Let's talk turkey. If you're used to running or biking 30 minutes to an hour, there is a chance you are inhibiting your immune system and you make you more susceptible to infections. The longer your work out, the more you make free radicals, and the more antioxidants your body is required to use. The antioxidants are going to support working out and not recovery, or more importantly, your immune system.

Instead of going hard for 30 minutes or an easy workout for an hour, perhaps change it to 15 to 20 minutes of HIT. What would it look like for a runner or somebody on an elliptical? I recommend 30 seconds fast-paced followed by 30 seconds slow-paced. Of course, one can change up their intervals such as 40/20, or one of my all-time favorites, which is a ladder. A ladder is 10 seconds hard, followed by10 seconds easy, followed by 20 seconds hard, then 20 seconds easy adding 10 seconds in duration to each interval up to a minute and back down. You don't have to go up to a minute. You might find it difficult in 30 seconds. Stop there! Don't hurt yourself in the process of trying to get healthy. These are fantastic boosts to your immune system and your cardiovascular system and your metabolic system and your brain.

What about different plans for different age groups? I mean, it's going to be hard to get a toddler to do high intensity training, so I would suggest you limit that to 12 years of age and older. But what about children younger than that? There's a myriad of activities that you can do such as jumping jacks, mountain climbers, running in place, or running from wall-to-wall. If you can go outside, and you have a fence at our yard boundary, run fence to fence in a shuttle run type of way.

I would not put too much emphasis on push-ups or sit-ups until they get to their preteen years. But I would make an emphasis for exercises that benefit the brain such as bridges, planks, and Superman. For brain function, you could benefit from these exercises too, not just your children.

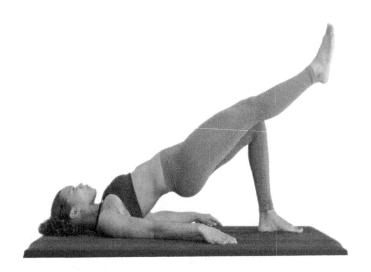

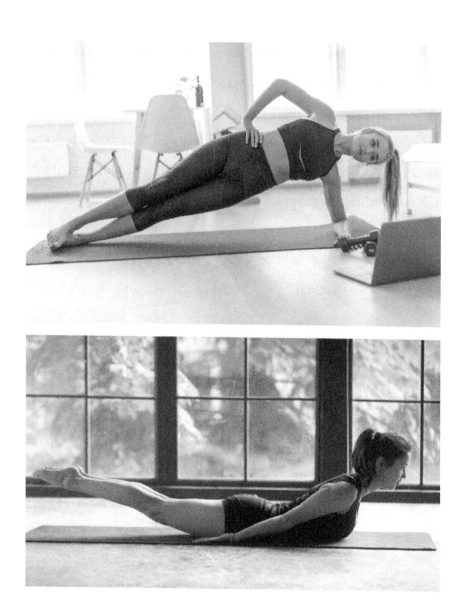

You can achieve this lesson 20 minutes today, or when things are going crazy at home, maybe you do this a couple times a day. Why not move and burn some energy up? If you're homeschooling or doing online learning, and that time is now limited, I would suggest you do your workout before your study.

The point of this is with some movement, HIT, or another home-based physical education, your children now have blood perfusing their brain where they can learn new skills to improve their memory faster. In our office, we were doing these things well before the pandemic so why can't you do them at home? You can and we want them to so your children have all the benefits for growth and health.

HIT vs easy to moderate workout

Goal of workout	HIT	Jogging/biking/intervals
Increase immunity	Best	Little
Reduce nociception	Best	None
Muscle growth	Best	None
eNOS	Best	Best
Blood sugar/insulin	Best	Little
Brain protection	Best	Best
ROS and excessive training risk	Best	Little

Another way to self-check yourself at home is to use a device that measures heart rate variability or HRV. Long story short, early detection can be achieved with routine morning HRV tracking. You need to know why heart rate variability is so important to you and your family.

A score of zero means there is no heartbeat. In the higher scores are important indicators of your health and are correlated to longevity and health. Another reason that is different from measuring heart rate is that a heart rate measuring device only provides you the average over time. For instance, HR is always in whole numbers, but if one minute I beat for 73 beats and the next minute I average seventy-two beats, then the average is 72 and half beats. HRV is an important indicator of health. Low heart rate variability is linked to heart disease and early death. HRV measures stress that you're unable to handle with normal functioning physiology. This includes heart rate, respiration, perspiration, and breathing. Regardless of its form from physical, chemical, mental, or emotional HRV shows you are under some form(s) of stress. The good news is you do have the ability to increase your HRV.

A long time ago, I got to work for the Nike Oregon track club, which was a group of elite track and field athletes who are Olympic hopefuls. We had a device that cost around $20,000 called the omega wave machine. With this device, we can measure the differences in the nervous system from stress or non-stress. From this information we would decide if their body was able to do a very hard workout or not. If they were not, we would change their workout to something easy until the athlete recovered.

We took this device to numerous cross-country camps and mapped thousands of kids to discover what was their best heart rate for working out. I follow the data we learned from these tests to get people to slow down. That could be those who are overworking, whether that is in their job or with exercise.

We found that most athletes benefited with recovery days using the heart rate of 150 beats per minute or less. We found that most individuals burn fat between 110 and 130 bpm, and athletes get to go up to 150 bpm. For whatever reason, when the heart rate gets above this, the body goes into a state of stress. The difference with this is measured with heart rate variability.

Unfortunately, the Omega wave machine is difficult and cumbersome to use because you must combine that with an EKG to measure the nervous system. Today, there is a device that your finger goes in for around $150 that can provide the same information that the Omega wave was doing.

There's a link to HRV testing at home for your family in the reference section. Most important, are you stressed or not, and how should your day respond with that information? And that brings us to the 5th subset (https://shortly.cc/sjMsz).

5. Life Quality-Stress Control

The fifth factor outside of supplements to boost your immune system is to live and enjoy life. When you're having fun through laughter and entertainment, you gain an opioid response. Opioids activate your T cells which improve immunity. This can happen through telling jokes, reading jokes, watching a funny movie, or catching up with a friend who makes you laugh.

Also, crying does have an opioid response, so if you have an emotional event that you've been harboring are having trouble working through, let it go. If you can't do it on your own, please get some professional help and talk it out.

Talking about an issue brings out an opioid response, which has a trigger to your brain to enhance your immune system. Holding issues in triggers a stress molecule and can slow down your immune system.

EFT

You can find many a funny chuckle online with our interactive world, but not always is there stress reduction or emotional health online. In the meantime, I'm going to provide you a link for a tapping technique called emotional freedom technique (EFT). This is not a replacement for proper care or counseling, but we know you can't go to a counselor every day. You can do EFT every day. Link is (https://www.emofree.com/)

For those of you here sitting around watching TV and waiting for the world to implode, I highly suggested using EFT. Again, if you are constantly thinking about a situation that is causing anxiety, these will decrease your opioids. A loss of opioids is not what you're shooting for.

Limit yourself on what you watch. Personally, I spend no more than 30 minutes on the news. Most of my time is research looking at clinical trials and breakthroughs so that I can bring that information to my clients. The rest of my time, I am looking for a solution we can do to prevent and decrease the negative effects of this pandemic.

The Stress Response

First, we need to understand how stress impacts your nervous system. A perceived acute stress can be worrying about exposure to a virus, a fight with a spouse, not sleeping, or eating inflammatory food. Acute stress triggers a cascade of hormones, neurotransmitters, and other chemicals that stimulate your fight or flight nervous system otherwise known as the sympathetic nervous system, (SNS.) When you're in a fight-or-flight mode, your body prioritizes energy and resources against a perceived threat. The other needs of your body are considered unnecessary such as digestion, sexual function, and other nonessential functions to fight infection or run away.

The important takeaway from this is that long periods of stress or major stresses can have a negative affect on your immune system. With HRV testing, one might notice a gradual decline in HRV scores in the morning. That can be an indicator that stress is increasing SNS, making it more active. If the SNS is overactive for too long, then your immune system can be compromised, leaving you vulnerable to illness, period. You can test your own HRV and that of your family at home with this home device that links to an individual device such as a phone or tablet. The one we recommend can be shared with any health care practitioner. You can decide if it's important for you to get a hard workout, push yourself, or it's time to see a doctor. [136] [137] [138] [139] [140] [141] [142] [143] [144] [145]

One major factor to help decrease the SNS pathway is adequate breathing. I'd like to share deep breathing skills that will build resilience towards stress with the ultimate goal of boosting your immune system and that of your family. The best use of that to increase your parasympathetic nervous system is to take 12 to 18 breaths per minute inhaling through your nose and out through your mouth. Compared to mouth breathing, slow diaphragmatic nasal breathing has benefits such as providing oxygen to the lower lungs which is embedded with parasympathetic nerve endings. It also provides nitric oxide, which is a bronchodilator and vasodilator that helps lower blood pressure and improve oxygen absorption. Also, it stimulates the vagus nerve which is the primary controller of your autonomic nervous system to balance both the SNS and the parasympathetic nervous system, or PNS.

In short, the right breathing stimulates your PNS, improves your mental state, and increases your HRV, all which help boost and support the immune system. In general, there are four steps to help with proper breathing, so let's get started. Take a deep breath through your nose, expanding your belly and not your chest or shoulders. Breathe out slower than you typically do, but not to the point of exertion, and exhaustion, or discomfort. First, take a deep breath through your nose with your lips closed. Try to breathe in as deep as you can. Then, put your tongue at the top of your mouth and purse your lips together and breath out. When you do this for 5-10 breaths and with deep breaths, you can stimulate the lower parts of your lungs, that have nerve endings to the parasympathetic nervous system. The PNS is tied into your immunity. So, work it out. Do this each day or more if you have many stressful events, or live in a stressful environment.

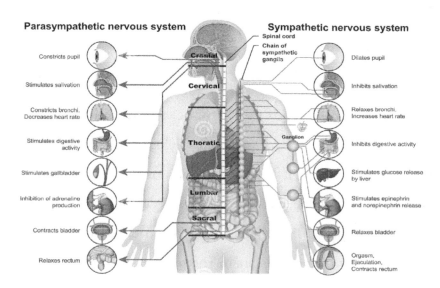

Blood types

I have read about concerns about blood types and illness susceptibility. It's true, certain blood types are more susceptible than others for certain diseases. That's genetics and expression. Unfortunately, there's no long-term study to substantiate current pandemics. However, there are a lot of studies that show that there are different immune reactions with different blood types and ethnicities.

So, while there is no long-term study that doesn't mean the blood type differences are ruled out, this new virus is affecting all blood types and all ethnicities. The reality is that there are many pathways for the immune system other than blood type.

Pandemics

It's time to address the elephant in the room, and that's world pandemic virus. I have written some articles about them, and that by no way makes me an expert, an epidemiologist or virologist. But I try to make sense of it and pass that information along. I'm sure you're aware that the COVID-19 virus breaks down lung tissue known as epithelial. Epithelial cells are a barrier cell that is also in your gut, sinuses, and your brain. The problem with this virus is it creates a leaky lung and you get pulmonary destruction from pneumonia.

Seemingly, the difference and degree of infection has to do with barrier issues. Barriers are your lungs, sinus, intestines, and brain. So, if you have barrier illnesses, you have a higher susceptibility. These include obesity, high blood pressure, asthma, liver disease, age, immunocompromised, diabetes, lung disease, kidney disease, and heart conditions. These all break down barriers and increase susceptibility.

There are other nutrients that can support or boost an immune system, and of course none have been studied in detail concerning COVID-19. The scary part of this disease is seemingly around day 10 when someone isn't getting better and their immune system creates a cytokine storm. The storm is a feedback loop where the immune system is running out of options and screaming for help.

In turn, there is an enormous release of these cytokine signals and everything in the immune system is activated to attack with reckless abandon. This creates an uncontrolled release of pro-inflammatory cytokines by the body's immune system as a result of this end stage viral infection. Meaning, your body is doing a Kamikaze attack on the virus at your expense. Cytokine storms and cytokine release syndrome can be activated with certain medications and other infections.

Currently, I am asked to explain what cytokines are. Roughly, they are signaling molecules in the immune system and they can be pro-inflammatory or actually good as anti-inflammatory. At some point, they need to turn the information off. They are kind of like a mass email or newsletter where you can sit down and individually email everyone on the list from one email.

Hormones act in a very similar way where one neurotransmitter tells thousands of hormones what to do. But a cytokine can be a million to one or more in their messaging. They're critical to your health and help cause a fever when exposed to an infection. When you cut yourself, they help you repair. But when you have long bouts of inflammation, or you eat a lot of inflammatory foods, or that couch has been held down for years, you can trigger the proinflammatory cytokines. If you have any interest in anti-aging and longevity and you do not want disease, make a change. Promote the anti-inflammatory cytokines because the inflammatory ones age you.

Cytokines have different names known as chemokines, interferons, interleukins, lymphokines, and tumor necrosis factor. They are generally not hormones or growth factors. Cytokines are produced by several types of cells including immune cells like B and T lymphocytes. A type of cytokine is not limited to be produced by one type of cell. They act through cell surface receptors and are especially important in the immune system. Cytokines modulate the balance between T1 and T2 immune responses, killer cells, and antibodies. They regulate growth and responsiveness of cell populations and are not limited to the immune system. Some cytokines enhance or down regulate the action of other cytokines in many ways. They are molecularly different from hormones, which are also important cell-signaling molecules. Hormones have higher concentrations in circulation and are made by specific kinds of cells, where cytokines can be made by different cells. Cytokines are important in health and disease. They help in immune responses to infection, inflammation, trauma, disease, and reproduction.

Cytokines single immune cells such as T cells and macrophages to go to the side of the infection where the immune system is fighting a pathogen. The signals activate those cells and stimulate them to reduce more cytokines. The feedback loop is managed by the body. But in some cases, it becomes unregulated with too many immune cells activating in a single location. This exaggerated immune response is not completely understood but could be attributed to the body encountering a new pathogenic attacker. The danger with cytokine storms is the potential to cause significant damage to various tissues and organs, especially if it attacks the lungs, macrophages, and fluids. This inflammatory response can obstruct the airway. I won't explain the intricacies of cytokines that are inflammatory and those that are anti-inflammatory. I will instead explain what foods and lifestyle options you have to create anti-inflammatory cytokines.

Immune Nutrition

You'll want to go through some trial and error to see what works best for you and your family. I also try not to dose or provide specific details on how to take them. That is between you and your doctor, the manufacturer, and how you feel taking them. In general, I would consider the manufactures dose from the label if I had nothing else to go with.

Antioxidants

Antioxidants are one of the best things to prevent issues. Foods that are high in sulfur such as asparagus, garlic, onion, and coconut help your body make antioxidants. N-acetyl cysteine, otherwise known as NAC, is a supplement to help make glutathione, one of the most powerful antioxidants that we know. Unfortunately, its rate is limited because glutathione can exasperate some asthmatic conditions, making them more susceptible to respiratory infections. So be careful with glutathione if you are asthmatic.[146] [147] [148] [149] [150] [151] [152] [153]

From a food standpoint, foods that are high in sulfur are important to the immune system. Considering the antioxidants are the most

169

important, the question is, will it protect the lung epithelial? Recently, I have witnessed quite a few smokers on the essential list on their way to work, or worse, outside of the hospital, yikes! If they haven't got the message, now is a good time to stop, because it decreases vitamin C, which is an antioxidant that supports epithelial tissue.

There are superfoods like acai, blueberry, and raspberry that are all high in antioxidants. We use them and other superfoods in our smoothies and shakes (https://shortly.cc/yB3uZ) . There is strong evidence for echinacea being useful for upper respiratory infections as well as elderberry in a capsule form, and not full of sugar as most liquids are. There is infant research on Japanese wormwood being specific for this condition, but again, each of us is unique and may not have the same response. None have been tested on new and emerging pandemics, but I will update as soon as the research is available on our website.

Fiber

One of the pathways requires getting enough fiber because it has short-chain fatty acids, which are the regulators of the immune system. A lot of Americans don't get enough fiber to support their immune system.

Where do you get fiber? Fruits and veggies. So, let's make a smoothie, right?

When you juice your food to a liquid, it eliminates the fiber and increases the carbohydrates. Without fiber and an increase in sugar, it is not beneficial to your immune system.

Short-chain fatty acids are parts of fiber that support the regulation of the immune system between the attacking portion and memory portion required for attacking future exposures. If you cannot digest fiber, it is important to consider a mashup program to get additional fiber. Butyrate is a fiber that is one of the best short chain fatty acids and helps support TH1, TH2, TH3 and TH17 pathways. [154]

Also, bacteria and your intestines are messenger protein producers and communicate with the immune system by a system called LPS. The more fiber you eat, the more the system communicates. The moral of this section is eat your veggies. Who knew? Which brings me to probiotics.[155] [156] [157]

Probiotics

In the past, almost everybody got a probiotic, and now every fruit, juice, and even milk have added probiotics. We've learned there are many variables to probiotics. There are different strains to help different conditions and ethnicities and genetic expression. So here is a rule for using a probiotic.

If there's a change in your symptoms for the better, than use that. If you don't feel better, or there's no changing some symptoms, then it may not be working for you.

Make sure that it comes in a DR gel capsule and does not need to be refrigerated.

It needs to have at least seven different strains with 15 billion cells at a minimum. That way you make sure it can get where it's supposed to go has enough power to make a difference.

Reduce Sugar

Also, keep your sugar to a minimum as it decreases your immune system. Be careful of foods that you have at home, because they could be full of inflammatory promoting foods. You will learn more about these foods.

Specific nutrients that can support portions of an immune system are:

Anti-Inflammatories

Outside of the coronavirus pandemic, there is evidence that curcumin, which comes from turmeric, can help mediate 150 of the cytokine signals. Anti-inflammatories are important for events such as a cytokine storm and in generalized pain in the body. Resveratrol, essential fatty acids, curcumin from turmeric, and Boswellia are natural anti-inflammatories.[158]

Barrier and Antioxidant

Barrier and major antioxidants consist of glutathione, NAC, and whey protein isolate because the latter can turn into glutathione. Resveratrol and turmeric are some of the biggest antioxidants after glutathione, followed by alpha lipoic acid, coQ10, ubiquinol, and other antioxidants. The thing with taking antioxidants is that you feel nothing and there isn't a blood test to say that there is a deficiency. There are several blood tests that show free radical damage, which antioxidants are to help reduce. Furthermore, there are not specific guidelines on how much to take. So, what we do now is eat or supplement as much as you can. So, if you eat no fruits or vegetables, you will need more supplements. If you have a disease state that causes inflammation and free radicals, you will need more antioxidants. Because dosing at best is a guess, you take as much as you can ingest and financially manage.[159] [160]

Fat-soluble Vitamins

Liquid vitamin D, K, A, and E are great ways to take these vitamins because they are all fat-soluble. All the rest of vitamins are water-soluble. When you take the fat-soluble vitamins and you take it with caffeine, it has a tendency to decrease your absorption. Do yourself a favor and take them away from products that contain caffeine. Again, there are no dosing specificities because all cases are different. What you do want is to get your vitamin D above 60, if not closer to 80, and get your blood test and your platelets to about 250. Most vitamin D labs have a reference range from 30 to 100. Anything between that is "normal." But the research shows above 60 is optimal pre-pandemic. But 80 appears to be viral protective, so we have increased our ranges on this new data.[161] [162] [163] [164]

Platelets are responsible for clotting. When they are low, you don't clot well. Should you take an Aspirin and other blood thinners, they don't thin your blood as you've been told. They bind to the platelet and make it less sticky. Then, you don't clot as well. For platelet response, you want your number to be above 250 on a scale and that is in general 150-450. Below, you may consider Vitamin K supplementation. K comes in several forms, K1, K2, K7. Choose a combination K unless you have a hereditary issue that you know of or your doctor has you on a blood thinner and K is a bad idea to add to your regiment. [165]

Good Fats

Essential fatty acids, Omega 3, EPA, and DHA are all types of good fats that support your immune system, brain, and nervous system. They're also anti-inflammatory compared and omega six which are in fried foods, grains, dairy, soy and other pro-inflammatory foods. There is a finger prick blood spot test that can measure your ratio between omega six and omega three fatty acids. (BRAIN SPAN LINK) The average American is 25 to 1 omega six to omega three. We want to be at a ratio 8:1 and what is considered perfect is 4:1. Again, there is no perfect dosing but speaking in generalities a standard dose is about 3 grams of essential fatty acids. Not all fatty acids are equal. They must have vitamin E to stabilize the fats from being oxidized or becoming rancid and detrimental.

Fat Digestion

Gall bladder support is important for those who have very low cholesterol, low vitamin D, low platelets, and/or a gallbladder that is inefficient or gone. Gallbladder support is important to be able to digest fats. Because vitamins A, D, E, and K are fat-soluble, some people are unable to absorb these without gallbladder support.

Blood Supply Support

Nitric oxide, oxygen, and blood circulation support are also important so that the blood supply can take the immune system to where it needs to work. There are multiple types of products that create nitric oxide, so you must be careful in what you choose. Products that have arginine or are derivatives of arginine, such as ED medications, can cause inflammation responses. These defeat the purpose. We only want products that create endothelial nitric oxide and not the neuronal or inflammatory nitric oxide that is in arginine. Vinpocetine, hepcidin, and the rind of the watermelon contains citrulline, products that support the correct nitric oxide endothelial pathway.[166] [167] [168] [169] [170]

Digestive Aids

Digestion support and oral tolerance support it important for those who have lost their oral tolerance, which means that they don't digest their foods. Physiology tells us when you don't digest your food or make the proper amount of saliva, you don't make the proper amount of stomach acid. When you lack acid, you don't fire with efficiency into your gallbladder or your pancreas. And when those do not fire right, you have undigested food arriving at your small intestine which causes inflammation, food sensitivities, and negative effects to your immune system. We have most of our patients start with an ounce of apple cider vinegar in the morning and then before meals. If there is no pain, then you qualify for digestion support. If you do have pain, you need to see a doctor. There could be an underlying issue such as an ulcer or bacterial infection known as Helicobacter pylori, the most common cause of ulcers.

Blood Sugar Handling

Blood sugar supplements can address both low and high blood sugar imbalances that need support. It doesn't matter which one you have, neither high nor low blood sugar is good. If you have elevated blood sugar, I would hope you're seeing a doctor.

If you were elevated but not confirmed diabetic, there are some products to consider. You may look into a rapid fast mimic diet followed by a long-term plan.[171] See our reference section for starters. If you're hypoglycemic, you need to eat more often throughout the day. Protein needs to be your first thing eaten in the morning. You may consider products that contain herbals and minerals such as Gymnema sylvestre, vanadium, and chromium to help stabilize blood sugar numbers.[172] [173] [174]

One of the fastest ways to raise your blood sugar is to eat carbohydrates. Carbohydrates defined means that they are fuel in the form of sugar that is not protein or fat. They're quick to be utilized for energy. Fat and protein can be converted into energy, but that requires energy to make that conversion. Not all carbohydrates are created equal. They are defined as whole carbohydrates and refined carbohydrates. The biggest difference is the amount of fiber it has. Fiber is rich in vitamins, minerals, and micro nutrients that are beneficial to your health.

Also, whole carbohydrates have a low glycemic index. This means that when you eat them, they don't raise blood sugar as fast as a refined or simple carbohydrates. But it still will to a certain degree. A few examples of some whole carbohydrates are sweet potatoes, beets, apples, pears, lentils, chickpea, and most legumes.

A refined carbohydrate has had all of the natural fiber stripped out and therefore cannot keep a blood sugar from spiking. Because there is a very rapid spike in blood sugar, there's also a very rapid crash. This leaves you shaky, irritable and now looking for a quick fix, which is more refined carbohydrates.

You can see how this becomes a roller coaster with ups and downs in blood sugar. It is very hard to stop once you're committed to refined carbohydrates. Food manufacturers are aware of this addiction, and that's why the vending machines are full of these products. Keep in mind refined carbohydrates have little to no nutritional value. Some examples of these are breads, pasta, white rice, pastries, potato chips, sodas, and candy. Roughly anything that contains high fructose corn syrup. If you want to kick your immune system in the butt and leave it vulnerable to infections and many other diseases, then eat some refined carbohydrates.

Intestinal Support

Gut support is also important because that is where the immune system assimilates. If you have a condition known as a leaky gut or have been told you have one, there is a lot more information than having a leaky gut. There are four different types of leaky gut and multiple factors that cause a leaky gut. It's best to know what type you have. In medical terms, a leaky gut is known as a permeable membrane. You need to understand the factors that trigger your leaky gut so that you can do your best to mitigate them. Those triggers and factors will be presented in another section, but it is warranted to work with somebody who understands these processes and can evaluate and test your triggers. You want a product that connects the membrane fibers and tightens up the gap junctions. These are the proteins that are broken down or lost, causing a permeable membrane. Your supplement needs research and publications regarding gap junctions. Otherwise, it's a high probability it has no value.[175] [176] [177] [178]

Allergies/Histamine Support

Histamine support may be required if you have systemic allergies, as allergies are inflammatory and breakdown barriers. Histamine causes in the intestines an influx of water, which leads to chronic diarrhea or loose stools. In the sinuses, you get drainage and post-nasal drip that can lead to a cough. While histamine is important, not managing it through diet and environmental awareness allows histamine to be inflammatory and bind up nutrients. These nutrients can be used in other parts of your immune system, like those that are necessary for fighting an infection. This is why I try to help as much as I can those who have allergies of any type. The bigger picture is they will have immune deficiencies elsewhere. Allergies in adults genetically makes sense. If you are over 50 years old and have a few genes that could be getting less efficient, and now you have allergies, that's normal.

Allergies in children are not normal. Their immune system is being challenged, and that needs to be addressed. Sometimes addressing with medications is necessary. Understand this. If you suppress the immune system, histamine, and don't attempt to address the why, there will be more medications and more allergies as they grow. There's growing research that most medications for allergies decrease the blood-brain barrier and over time cause a leaky brain. By taking these at an early age, it increases brain breakdown, inflammation, and digestive disorders. Long term use of over-the-counter antihistamines is very scary. In fact, for every year you take them, the probability of dementia goes up.

179 180 181

Minerals

Minerals such as zinc and magnesium are important in many parts of the immune system. For most of my clients, they take Epsom salt foot baths to get the most amount of magnesium into their system. Magnesium is required for over 300 enzymatic pathways and is important for detoxification. When you do an Epsom salt bath, you need to have one cup of Epsom salt in a small tub of water that only your feet can fit in, or four cups in a tub where your body soaks. The water needs to be as hot as you can tolerate but not enough to scald you, and less hot for a child. Aim to be in the bath for about 15 minutes.[182] [183]

Home Testing for Quality and Function

While many of these supplements are great, some are not perfect for everyone. An easy test is called a pulse test. If you take, eat, breathe in a new environment, you may want to check your pulse. There are a lot of devices that take it for you so it's easier than looking at your watch and counting. If you eat or ingest anything, your pulse shouldn't change more than 10 beats per minute. So, if you are sitting at 60, anything under 70 is normal following ingesting. If you go, say to 75 beats per minute after eating eggs, you may have an issue with eggs or any other product or food you are testing. The same could be said for any pill you take. Blood pressure, temperature, and heart rate will all change with reactions. I bring this to your attention now for you and some autoimmune cases. We see it so often. Even very healthy foods can cause inflammation because a food or supplement is acting upon one side of their immune system.

In recap, before you reach for a whole bunch of supplements, make sure that you have adequate sleep, that you are hydrating enough. That you enjoy what you can, working on yourself, moving, and exercising. And of course, you know this, do not binge watch TV, stay up too late, and eat whatever.

If you like, you can send your email to marketing@newleafhealthandwellness.com, and you will receive a link to a company called Full Script. They sell for hundreds of supplement companies. On their website is a template that I've created that you will get specific for nutrients that are known to support the immune system. Is it perfect? Absolutely not. Will I add to it? Yes. But if you don't have the time, finances, or the ability to go learn all that you can, here's a fantastic shortcut that you can help yourself and your family keep your immune system as efficient as possible.

CHAPTER 7

Autoimmunity

Did you know that over 50 million Americans have an autoimmune disease and yet nearly 48 million are unaware? Why? Because doctors don't always do the necessary testing or they may not be aware of such tests being available.[184]

Autoimmunity is a condition where the body attacks itself. There are several ways in which this occurs. First, the body can make antibodies to itself, and this leads to tissue destruction. Second, the body can up-regulate white blood cells that can actually attack and destroy tissue. [185]

All of these are done through cellular communication and signaling that has gone awry. This happens for a myriad of reasons. Genetics is a big concern. If you have someone in your family with an autoimmune disease, the incidence of you having one is high. There is a high probability those you are related to are also gluten intolerant, whether they know it or not. Thus, the body produces antibodies to a specific tissue or the macrophages go in to destroy the tissue.

There are a lot of reasons for genetics to create autoimmunity. Some of these causes are internal such as hormonal changes, immune deficiencies, and infections. Others can be live, pollutants, reactive dietary proteins, food allergies, and life stresses. These could be from work and/or relationships yet all lead to what is called immune dysregulation. Over time this becomes a loss of self-regulation and self-tolerance. If you are gluten intolerant, it unfortunately was genetic. After symptoms come up, a few tests are run to confirm or deny its presence.It can also affect your brain and you appear drunk, uncoordinated and have brain fog.[186] [187] [188]

Often, the diagnosis of autoimmune disease is given. These conditions have names such as Graves, Hashimoto's thyroiditis, psoriatic arthritis, diabetes, muscular dystrophy, and lupus, although there are many more. This means a lifetime of treatment and management. Autoimmunity is an incurable disease.[189] [190] [191] [192]

Have you been diagnosed with an autoimmune disease, leaky gut, permeable membrane, or brain fog? If you have a leaky gut, autoimmune disease so much begins in the gut with the breakdown between your small intestine and large intestine. This is where the majority of your immune system lies.

If you do have a leaky gut or permeable membrane, it's important to understand what type. Are you paracellular or transcellular, do you or do you not have endotoxemia? Have you had traumatic brain injuries, or concussions? All these add to or take away from your outcome, and recovery.

There are multiple ways to address autoimmune conditions. Conventional treatment consists of medication and that's about it. It's about management and there is no true long-term solution other than increasing your dosage. For most people with autoimmune conditions, or who think they may have one, this isn't your only choice. Those whose tissues are destroyed by their autoimmune disease may never recover. But they can have a better outlook on life by making some important changes.

Autoimmune disease can have many facets allowing it to run rampant. Blood sugar handling, infections, chemical toxins and pollutants can all turn on autoimmune genes. First, the body can make antibodies to itself, and this leads to tissue destruction. Second, the body can up-regulate white blood cells that can actually attack and destroy tissue.

All of these are done through cellular communication and signaling that has gone awry, those pesky cytokines. This happens from many possibilities from before. Any one of these can over or under activate the two pathways for immunity, even if it's immune to yourself. That is what AI is.[193] [194] [195] [196] [197] [198] [199] [200] [201] [202]

You may have a leaking gut, otherwise known in medical literature as intestinal permeability. Over 200 clinical papers have been published on this topic on PubMed. A leaky gut can be a hindrance to recovery or a precursor to autoimmunity. That means it's a real thing, not something made up by alternative doctors. Our office uses laboratory testing to show how long your treatment plan should be and how to address this inflammatory condition. It is also to confirm an autoimmune condition and/or leaky gut and what stage you are in. [203] [204]

Below is just a few of the ways you can create a intestinal permeability but this is not the only options. There are more. Emotional (EMO) stress, genetically modified foods (GMO,) traumatic brain injuries (TBI,) high blood sugar (AGE's,), autoimmunity (AI,) neurodegeneration (ND,) and gastrointestinal (GI) inflammation. And how many ways are there to acquire these? The ways are infinite.

Stress	Chemical-environment meds heavy metals	Diet	Infection	Hormonal	Neuro	Metabolic
Life	Steroids	Gluten	SIBO	Low hormones	TBI	AGE's
Mental	Antibiotics	Casein	Bacterial	Thyroid	Concussion	AI
EMO	Anti-acids	GMO	Viral	Extra/inc thyroid hormones	Stroke	GI inflammation
Chem	Hormone replacement	Junk food	Parasite		ND	
Physical		Alcohol				

Regarding your immune system, it is run neurologically by the parasympathetic nervous system (PNS). This system is responsible for urination, defecation, procreation, digestion, and immunity. This is why most autoimmune patients have difficulty in these areas. It's all connected. While one can take supplements or medication, it is unfortunate that rarely do any oral recommendations have an effect on your parasympathetic nervous system. It is more important than balance, exercise, slow movement, gargling, self-gagging, and even coffee enemas. The combination movement is to connect the musculature, organs, and nervous system. So balance and PNS exercise are vital to your recovery and management.

The most important thing you can do for your nervous system is to maintain some form of structure mechanoreceptor treatments. I inform you of this because the literature has study after study how this slows down autoimmunity. You would be shocked to find out how influencing a balanced pelvis or muscles in the neck are upon the nervous system, thus dampening leaky gut and autoimmune conditions. In fact, there are articles on PubMed that show this may be even more beneficial than nutrition and diet alone!

Most structural physicians may need 2-3 visits a week and then slow down to weekly after a month or so. That's a lot of time and money. Is there something you can do for yourself? Yes. To be covered at the end of this book. I know in the beginning, when one is very inflamed, 2-4 times a month is adequate. I'll digress to what the literature states. Because of the profound effect of the immune system communicating with the nervous system, the best outcome for a structure based visit is four weeks once you are out of a crisis mode. Crisis mode could be symptomatic as you're in a lot of pain or can't remember anything, or your blood tests are confirming a condition and inflammation is running rampant. As you start to feel better, you can slow down mechanoreceptor/structure treatments. But please do not omit them if you're autoimmune. Here's why. After about four weeks, autoimmune tissue begins to decay and cause inflammatory issues. Joint destruction begins at 8 weeks. After this, you lose the momentum gained. I encourage my AI patients to come in no longer than 12 weeks. Otherwise, you're starting over on your recovery and maintenance. This is so detailed in the literature, and people put effort out for a bit, then either change doctors or stop the plan. I want you to understand the importance of structure mechanoreceptor stimulation. At home, I recommend some of the reference tools in Chapter 13. It's a big bang for a little buck. Or, you can see a massage therapist, chiropractor, physical therapist, or other person who physically stimulates your nervous system.

Genetics is a big concern for most individuals. If you've been searching for health, DNA testing should be a step in your journey. If you're already seeing an FM doctor and working on your autoimmunity, then genetic testing should be your next step. If you have someone in your family with an autoimmune disease, then the chances of you having one it goes up. [205]

Then it gets more disappointing. If you have an autoimmune disease, the probability of another autoimmune disease is a probability. It's called poly-autoimmunity. If you don't completely understand that concept, you're not alone. Most doctors don't. You need to be a physician to understand the mechanisms, or at least try to understand what allowed you to get to this point. Below are cross reactant antibodies for proper testing of poly-autoimmunity.

| TEST | RESULT | | | |
Array 5 – Multiple Autoimmune Reactivity Screen **	IN RANGE (Normal)	EQUIVOCAL*	OUT OF RANGE	REFERENCE (ELISA Index)
Parietal Cell + ATPase	0.98			0.1-1.4
Intrinsic Factor	0.34			0.1-1.2
ASCA + ANCA		1.25		0.2-1.4
Tropomyosin	1.13			0.1-1.5
Thyroglobulin	0.85			0.1-1.3
Thyroid Peroxidase	0.92			0.1-1.3
21-Hydroxylase (Adrenal Cortex)		1.02		0.2-1.2
Myocardial Peptide	0.97			0.1-1.5
Alpha-Myosin	0.96			0.3-1.5
Phospholipid			2.34	0.2-1.3
Platelet Glycoprotein	0.62			0.1-1.3
Ovary/Testis ***		0.94		0.1-1.2
Fibulin	1.19			0.4-1.6
Collagen Complex			1.88	0.2-1.6
Arthritic Peptide		1.03		0.2-1.3
Osteocyte		1.18		0.1-1.4
Cytochrome P450 (Hepatocyte)		1.47		0.3-1.6
Insulin + Islet Cell			2.88	0.4-1.7
Glutamic Acid Decarboxylase 65	1.19			0.2-1.6
Myelin Basic Protein		1.15		0.1-1.4
Asialoganglioside	0.75			0.1-1.4
Alpha-Tubulin + Beta-Tubulin	0.92			0.4-1.4
Cerebellar			1.48	0.2-1.4
Synapsin	0.78			0.1-1.2

What can your doctor do for you? First, one needs to know if they actually have said condition, and if you know you do see how prolific it is. A series of tests should be run for antibodies and tests to assure the tests are valid. Second, once that is discovered and you have a positive, what caused it? Will you need to be with a medical doctor, can your natural physician dampen the response with a change in diet, lifestyle, and immune system support? This all leads to be seen once you've been diagnosed and what the true prognosis will be. A natural physician is not your end-all or curative agent. If they're not looking at blood sugar, stress, sleep, and diet as we already spoke as preventative measures, are you in the right place?

Most of the time in the beginning, chances are you'll feel better about your condition regardless of therapy. The reality is your autoimmune disease is advancing without slowing your disease process. Most of the time you'll have your auto-immune antibodies for the rest of your life. That said, some patients respond in such a way where they don't look like they ever had a problem to begin with.

There are several levels with autoimmunity. If you have an antibody, it does not mean you have a disease. First, it has to meet and go beyond the reference ranges. That is called stage one. Second, it would be helpful for diagnostic purposes to have symptoms. Combine that with antibodies and that's stage two. And last in order, to be called autoimmune, there needs to be tissue destruction. This is generally proven through biopsy and pathological examination. Now this is stage three. If you have symptoms, but your antibody level isn't high enough and/or your tissue destruction isn't existent, be thankful. Congratulations, you don't have a diagnosable autoimmune disease, yet. In all probability, you're on your way. What can you do to slow it down naturally? First, manage your blood sugar handling. Second, watch your food intake. You don't want inflammatory foods. Third, support your immune system from the previous chapter. Fourth, regulate toxins. Fifth, support your brain. Last, support with supplements.[206]

Research literature continues to point to the previous paragraph to keep your family well. Yes, there are tweaks specific to each case and condition. But that's my point. Most of us do not do enough to support blood sugar, digestion, inflammation, and other fundamental issues. It's not always that simple, but it's an enormous step.

Over the past 19 years, I have tested more and more individuals for gluten sensitivity. Before you put the book down thinking you have to get rid of everything you love to eat, there is a difference between gluten sensitivity, gluten intolerance, and celiac disease. Let's start with the worst disease case, celiac disease. In order to be clinical, one needs to have one of two gene phenotypes: HLA DQ2 or HLADQ8. Antibodies can be measured in the blood, gluten antibodies, and the transglutaminase antibody. Then you need a tissue biopsy for true confirmation. Then and only then they are considered celiac. But you could have symptoms of celiac, or even no symptoms at all.

I will define that gluten sensitivity is not the same as a severe allergy. When tested, it does not show positive on a skin scratch test or for a particular antibody that is responsible for anaphylaxis. This is a severe and life-threatening immune reaction, IgE, for when people carry an Epi-Pen. [207] [208] [209]

One must have further testing to see if they are gluten sensitive. If so, I order an array of testing for foods that also may look like gluten to a body that is affected. Although a gluten sensitivity isn't celiac, that causes that pathophysiological destruction. It can lead to nervous system dysfunction, especially in the brain by creating inflammation here. It attacks the brain more than other tissues in the body. Although, the pancreas, skin, heart, liver, and digestive system aren't off limits. [210]

What is more frustrating, most gluten sensitivity doesn't have much to do with gastrointestinal symptoms. Why? Because there isn't much nociception or pain receptors in the bowel. The nervous tissue goes to a part in the brain more related to emotions ,and why with gluten sensitivity individuals can have anxiety and or depression. Nociception is pain receptors and goes to a different part of the brain. This is why the literature shows that around 60 percent of gluten sensitivity individuals have no gastrointestinal complaints. Chew on that for a bit.[211]

194

Moreover, wheat has been genetically modified. It changed from where it once was with a complex carbohydrate and its protein gluten and much more. I recommend reading Wheat Belly [212] to learn the history of wheat changes. And why gluten, in the presence of sugar intake and stress, of all kinds, can create gluten sensitivity and autoimmunity. Once you've taken the time to thumb through that, I recommend another book, Grain Brain, to learn a Neurologist's perspective on gluten. [213]It includes his first hand evaluation of neurological disorders that have responded to no medical intervention, but instead to gluten sensitivity and education on what is the best management for his patients. For both of these books, I have observed much they speak about and found alternative references during my own investigation. Last, I recommend www.glutenfreesociety.org, a free reference website and also in our reference section below.

In those with gluten sensitivities, only one-third have intestinal issues. Yup, you read that right. All you have to do now is turn on the television and you can hear a commercial asking you to get tested for other symptoms. Gluten sensitivities affect other tissues such as the brain, thyroid, pancreas, skin, joints and nervous system. This is more important when compared to celiac. Most of us know the main sources of gluten: wheat, spelt, oats, and barley. There are hidden sources such as modified food starch, dextrin, transglutaminase in meat glue, and meat tenderizer, malt extract, shampoo, cosmetics, and glue. And they can cross react with milk, whey, oats, sesame, corn, and yeast that are packed gluten-free. This is why gluten education is paramount. [214] [215]

For a large percentage of my patients ,they avoid gluten, manage blood sugar, and although they feel better, they still don't feel 100 percent. Why? Cross-reactive foods. A cross reactant is one of the most difficult concepts to explain in my office. How can something like milk act like gluten, I'm asked? I explain it by putting my hands together with my fingers interlocked. The left hand is gluten, and the right hand is a gluten specific antibody. If you flip your hand, or even remove a finger or two you can still interlock, or bind hands. From an immune standpoint you still get the same result, inflammation, and over time tissue destruction. So, you can be gluten-free and your body is not responding as if it's gluten-free. That sucks and I have calculated it happens 25% of the time. [216] [217] [218] [219] [220] [221]

If you're curious what you may be reacting to, I recommend going to the only lab I am comfortable in utilizing, Cyrex. It's the only lab I know that has this technology. And can make a world of difference in the management of those with these particular inflammatory conditions. Not managing what you are cross reacting to can continue your gluten sensitivity and your inflammatory pathway. There is always a chance if you've taken steps to help your condition and now you've dampened your autoimmunity. Now, if any tests run came back negative. That's called remission. Or even if you did everything you could, your immune system could still be on the verge of destruction,

This is the reason we use Cyrex labs. There is so much that occurs in physiology with autoimmunity conditions. In the case of gluten sensitivity, a main mechanism is the DPP IV enzyme. This enzyme is involved in the degradation of proteins such as gliadin and casein, a product of milk. DPP IV helps support the immune system. Also, you need brush border enzymes such as amylase, invertase, and lactase. These are your main gut enzymes. They support the digestion of carbohydrates, proteins, and fat without causing irritation and digestion of the intestinal walls. Without the brush border, you have intestinal permeability, or more well-known on the internet as leaky gut.[222] [223] [224] [225]

Finally, key antioxidants have been shown to help intestinal response. These are glutathione and fat-soluble vitamins A and D. You can order a Cyrex test for gluten cross reactants, polymorphic antibodies, mucosal antibodies, and food sensitivities on our website. Below are cross reactants to wheat and the intestine.

Array 3 – Wheat/Gluten Proteome Reactivity & Autoimmunity	IN RANGE (Normal)	EQUIVOCAL*	OUT OF RANGE	REFERENCE (ELISA Index)
Wheat IgG	0.82			0.3-1.5
Wheat IgA	0.22			0.1-1.2
Wheat Germ Agglutinin IgG	0.62			0.4-1.3
Wheat Germ Agglutinin IgA	<0.20			0.2-1.1
Native & Deamidated Gliadin 33 IgG	0.25			0.2-1.2
Native & Deamidated Gliadin 33 IgA	0.23			0.1-1.1
Alpha Gliadin 17-mer IgG	0.78			0.1-1.5
Alpha Gliadin 17-mer IgA	0.17			0.1-1.1
Gamma Gliadin 15-mer IgG	1.05			0.5-1.5
Gamma Gliadin 15-mer IgA	0.19			0.1-1.0
Omega Gliadin 17-mer IgG	0.70			0.3-1.2
Omega Gliadin 17-mer IgA	0.37			0.1-1.2
Glutenin 21-mer IgG			2.05	0.1-1.5
Glutenin 21-mer IgA	0.26			0.1-1.3
Gluteomorphin + Prodynorphin IgG	0.72			0.3-1.2
Gluteomorphin + Prodynorphin IgA	0.31			0.1-1.2
Gliadin-Transglutaminase Complex IgG	0.48			0.3-1.4
Gliadin-Transglutaminase Complex IgA	0.22			0.2-1.5
Transglutaminase-2 IgG	0.94			0.3-1.6
Transglutaminase-2 IgA	0.35			0.1-1.6
Transglutaminase-3 IgG	0.78			0.2-1.6
Transglutaminase-3 IgA			1.55	0.1-1.5
Transglutaminase-6 IgG	0.63			0.2-1.5
Transglutaminase-6 IgA	0.48			0.1-1.5

Autoimmune Management and Rules to Follow:

So, what causes the body, if you don't have an all-out genetic response, to have an issue? Many times, it can be attributed to the concept of intestinal permeability or leaky gut. The mechanisms of a leaky gut consist of diets high in sugar, gluten, infections, yeast overgrowth, and stress that creates a spike in cytokines (inflammatory cellular receptors) cortisol. It could also be hormonal changes, many medications, antibiotic usage, neurological disorders, and metabolic dysfunctions to name a few.

Now, because you've had one of these, does it mean you have a leaky gut? No. Remember, it's all about how your body handles the load. A select group of folks are gifted with genetics. They can drink copious amounts of alcohol, smoke, eat bacon, fast food, drink liters of cola, and somehow thrive. It's my understanding they have superior glutathione handling, methylation, and recycling.

Unfortunately, that's not the majority of us, and especially those who end up in my office wondering why they feel the way they do. Or, autoimmunity has not been explained to them. Most patients don't understand that once they have the issue, the likelihood of their tissues breaking down increases over time. Even more so with life events or stressors. What type or types of permeable membrane do you have? Are there infections, heavy metals, immune complexes and some of the main food allergies that cause this involved? What about some autoimmune markers specific to the intestine? For this we prefer to run a Cyrex Array 14 salivary test for multiple mucosal immune reactivity. Below is an example of this test with green being good and red very reactive.

Array 14 - Multiple Mucosal Immune Reactivity Screen	IN RANGE (Normal)	EQUIVOCAL*	OUT OF RANGE	REFERENCE (ELISA Index)
Total Secretory IgA		2.78		0.0-3.0
Lipopolysaccharides IgA+IgM			>2.90	0.0-2.6
Occludin/Zonulin IgA+IgM			>4.30	0.0-2.3
Actomyosin IgA+IgM			>6.10	0.0-3.3
ASCA/ANCA IgA+IgM			>3.80	0.0-2.4
Calprotectin IgA+IgM	1.17			0.0-3.1
Alpha-Gliadin-33-mer IgA+IgM			2.44	0.2-2.0
Gamma-Gliadin-15-mer IgA+IgM			>4.30	0.0-3.1
Glutenin-21-mer IgA+IgM	1.45			0.0-2.6
Gluteomorphin IgA+IgM			>3.60	0.0-2.5
Wheat Germ Agglutinin IgA+IgM		2.79		0.0-3.6
Transglutaminase 2 IgA+IgM			3.23	0.0-3.1
Egg IgA+IgM			3.90	0.0-2.7
Soy IgA+IgM			2.07	0.2-2.0
Corn IgA+IgM			2.64	0.2-2.3
Alpha + Beta Casein IgA+IgM		2.17		0.0-2.6
Casomorphin IgA+IgM	1.61			0.0-2.5
Aflatoxin IgA+IgM			3.46	0.0-3.4
Bisphenol-A IgA+IgM			2.23	0.2-2.2
Mercury IgA+IgM			6.47	0.0-4.4
Mixed Heavy Metals IgA+IgM			>5.40	0.0-3.4
Rotavirus IgA+IgM			3.25	0.0-2.5
Myelin Basic Protein IgA+IgM			4.48	0.0-3.2
Blood-Brain Barrier Proteins IgA+IgM			4.99	0.0-3.6
Immune Complexes IgA+IgM			3.02	0.0-2.9

Over 70 percent of the human body's immune cells are found in the gut's mucosal lining. A healthy gut leads to more immunity, and in most cases, this means the healthy bacteria outnumbers the bad. In fact, our bowels can explain your current health situations with good accuracy. You should be tested for any gastrointestinal complaint through stool testing. Why aren't doctors testing this? Well, most doctors don't appreciate a patient bringing a stool sample into the office. Most doctors don't know they can send it out.

For years, I didn't do stool testing, because from my time in the laboratory, stools were sent in through small coffee-tin-like containers. Then summer comes around. UPS, FedEx, and other carriers deliver the end product. Many times, that means leaving these ready to explode ticking time bombs containers on the loading dock, ever expanding. Guess what we did in the lab when these time bombs came in? Rock, paper, scissor, shoot. When you see the dents in the canister, we first cursed the carrier for delivering it outside, then the ordering physician for making our life hell. Then, we have to gown up and muster up the courage to pry this little delicatessen lid open. That, of course, after a quick prayer to the almighty that it won't explode all over you and the room, leaving much to curiosity.

When it did happen, and it did, questions arose in my head such as, How bad am I contaminated? I mean, they ordered this test right for a reason, right? Am I going to die? What did this person have? Did I clean it all off me? Should I burn my clothes, even though I had a lab coat on? Thank goodness for vented hoods, gloves, and face masks. For years, thinking back to my lab days, I couldn't find it in me to re-order those tests. Well, I'm over it, and I was able to leave the field in pursuit of a less messy career.

Now, we can have you take a sample at home and they don't come in tin cans. Most are on paper. And, they can measure your microbiome. The microbiome is all the cells in your body that are not you. They are not human. You have yeast, bacteria, viruses, parasites, fungus, and mold living in you. Some are disease causing and pathogenic, others are beneficial. A stool sample can test what percentage of good and bad bacteria you have in your intestines. If you have too many bad bacteria, the lab can also run tests to see if they are sensitive. This means they can kill what shouldn't be there either with antibiotics or natural antibiotics, such as garlic or oregano. Also, microbiome gut testing tells us what food to eat and what food does not support our gut based on genetic expression. How cool![226] [227]

If your doctor isn't asking you about bowel movements and you're not having at least three a day, there could be something missing in your evaluation and require testing. In case you didn't know, sinus congestion, acne, itching, eczema, hives, rashes, belching, heartburn, bad breath, asthma, ADD/ADHD are all signs of bowel issues.

If you have used antibiotics, antacid, probiotics, traveled outside the country, eat GMO foods, and have any history of gastritis and ulcers, you qualify for a stool test. That doesn't lead to very many folks in the U.S. at this point. Can you see why we may have concerns with our food and medications? To your body, manufactured products are not seen as food. [228]

Autoimmune Triggers

Manufactured food, GMOs, have been shown to transfer their genetic material into the DNA of bacteria in the intestinal tract lining. This causes many health issues. The American Academy of Environmental Medicine has warned against its use and stated there are "Serious health risks. These include infertility, decreased immunity, antibiotic resistant infections, and poor insulin regulation." Even the animals we may eat that consume GMO foods can pass some of these properties onto us.

When we have intestinal permeability, as well as several other conditions, we can lose our tolerance to many things. Often, out of the blue, we become intolerant to smells, metals on our body, shampoo, lotions, detergents, and foods. This leads to skin outbreaks and lots and lots of frustration. This is how someone can do a heavy metal hair analysis and it comes back positive. After treatment, those folks may not be better, or worse, they are indeed worse. Many doctors tell them they must get worse to get better, or they're having a healing crisis. I'm alternative minded, but this is absolute nonsense. If that happens in my office, we stop because either I didn't ask something or I wasn't told something. Like recently, "Oh yeah, doc. I didn't put this on my intake or tell you. I'm celiac and so is my entire family!"

Or there's something no one understood and this is a new reaction. It could be a physiological change that wasn't investigated or understood. It could even mean that I wasn't aware of this possibility for a reaction and it's tough to swallow.

No, I'm not perfect and that's clear. Luckily, this is a probable, very low percentage in my patient population, and when it does, I go into research mode. Yes, this sounds somewhat sadistic. But when I have a patient not responding to what so many do, I now have an opportunity to learn and grow. When you're pushed and you get through it, have you ever looked back on how much you've learned?

I speak of this knowing what I have been taught and what I've retained through learning. When I didn't get an educated result, I wondered if I was a dunce, or I didn't get the concept, or the mechanism. Or, even worse, my $1,000,000 education hadn't exposed me to something. More often than not, it was the latter and I needed to learn more. I estimate a person can spend their entire life in their field of expertise and at the end say, "I may know 1%."

Gut permeability has other causes than eating too much sugar or having a love-hate relationship with another person. It could be from infections or other sources of stress, such as brain trauma and even body trauma, or chronic sources of inflammation such as poor sleep and poor sleep habits.

Or, malnutrition can lead to a loss of the immune system, which in itself has a limited tolerance for chemicals that we are exposed to on a daily basis.

Once we have lost our tolerance, we are either depleted in our glutathione, or we can no longer recycle it, leading to an increase or build-up of toxicity. The cellular function of our immune cells, especially those known as T-cells, are no longer regulated. Without this, we get inflammatory hormones running rampant. This is the beginning of food and chemical sensitivities.

Once you've gotten to this point, you're pretty far down the road. It's not an overnight fix, unless it recently occurred. Sometimes this happens with exposure to high doses of mercury or radiation. If the damage isn't too great, you may recover quickly. But that is rare. Once your T-Cells are unregulated, the symptoms come. These are fatigue, persistent pain from inflammation, tissue breakdown and degeneration. You may even have a long or chronic illness, and even, dare I say it, autoimmunity. This condition is also known as toxic induced loss of tolerance or (TILT.)

When someone comes into my office, we educate on how to be proactive about their lives. We look at where they live, work, sleep, eat, workout, and how they breathe. There's a lot of literature that can at times be overwhelming.

If I walk, run, or bike outside during peak rush hour, will I be exposed to pollution? How much sunscreen is safe, and what is toxic? How cooked does the food need to be before it's considered overdone, charred, or toxic? Where do I get my water? Should it be filtered, well, plastic bottle, or aluminum container? How should I store my food? Is the food I buy toxic? Are the cosmetics, lotions, potions ,and creams I put on adding to my load? Should I go native and live in a cave?

First, I ask, does the cave have mold, adequate ventilation, access to sunlight, clean drinking water? I digress. All this doesn't matter, yet. What matters is how a person can clean up their system. Do they have a good recycling system? Do they have adequate glutathione available to handle life as it is? Or if in panic mode, the dangers of cave living?

The only way I can answer this is to test. I can tell you this from experience. If you're having symptoms, there's a high degree of certainty that either you've depleted your glutathione or your recycling system is inadequate. In that case, we need to see why. And if it's so bad that you cannot stop your body from attacking itself, or worse, cause further inflammation, we start going into the details of lifestyle management so you can begin to feel well again.

I'll take a few moments to go through other necessary functions of glutathione. We've gone over the fact that it's a wonderful antioxidant and it grabs those toxic free radicals and becomes oxidized, rendering it useless. For most antioxidants, this is the end of the road. They are packaged and excreted from the body. Glutathione can be converted back to a working agent. By a recycling pathway using the enzyme glutathione reductase, it can go grab the next free radical.

As we age, our bodies decrease our digestive ability. Often, we begin taking proton pump inhibitors. When we take these or antacids, we can no longer absorb enough of our protein. This will also decrease our ability to create the enzyme, as those are protein molecules. Perhaps reducing our ability to be efficient with recycling glutathione. Yes, getting older can suck, and life happens.

But knowing what to do and prevention is paramount to your success in anti-aging.

From a medical model, this is a hard one to "fix" or manage. For a patient who is prescribed antacids or other proton pump inhibitors, they now have a side effect of decreased protein digestion. These cause constipation and malabsorption because the undigested proteins cannot cross the brush border in the gut.

Glutathione is also involved in energy production by supporting the mitochondria, the power houses of every cell. The mitochondria are responsible for making our life protein, adenosine triphosphate (ATP). In the lung, N-acetyl cysteine is converted to glutathione and supports the lung-epithelial barrier. And in the gut, it supports the intestinal barrier needed to prevent intestinal permeability, or leaky gut.

More importantly, glutathione supports the blood brain barrier. This is responsible for keeping our brain from being exposed to toxins and infections. In the liver, it helps break down solids to liquids so they can be excreted. It also supports nitric oxide balance, the good endothelial one. For your immune system, it helps support proper T-cell function. Glutathione is important, don't you think?

If your physician isn't asking you questions about all of those systems, I disagree. How can they be adequate in your treatment? And if they are holistic and aren't asking these, they have a completely different set of values. It could be a case of wishful thinking, arrogance, laziness, or ignorance. I understand many doctors treat the patients' complaints, but I have to ask why, what, where, when, and how? What else could it be? When could the next phase come in? Is it a new set of symptoms, or do we need advanced laboratory testing? If I don't test for it, chances are patients will find someone who will. Even if it's the wrong test or not a functional test.

For instance, I use thyroid stimulating hormone (TSH) to strengthen my point. I've witnessed hundreds of physicians and life-insurance companies testing this hormone alone to tell a patient their thyroid is good. As I sit here shaking my head, TSH is not a thyroid hormone. It's actually a pituitary hormone that attempts to guide the thyroid into making thyroid hormone in two subsets, T4 and T3. T4 is then converted in the liver and the gastrointestinal system. A part of the brain, the hypothalamus, reads the number of T3 and T4 not used and sends its hormone for thyroid to the pituitary. Now, the pituitary will increase or decrease the release of TSH levels. And, there are seemingly an infinite amount of exposures and lifestyles choices that influence these levels. [229] [230] [231] [232] [233] [234] [235]

THYROID CASCADE

TSH from **Pituitary**

Thyroid Releasing hormone from
Hypothalamus

Thyroid making T3* and T4**
*most biologically active
*93% of thyroid hormone made

Liver uses 5' diodinase enzyme to convert T4 to T3

Intestines have bacteria to convert T4 to T4

Again, if you're not able to absorb protein because of age, brain health, or antacids, this affects TSH levels as it is a hormone. And hormones are made of cholesterol, which is transported by proteins. Can the levels go down if you're measuring TSH and not the other

210

hormones or players in this cycle? You bet. What if the T4 isn't being converted in the liver?

The hypothalamus signals bring the TSH down because there's plenty of T4. So, you would appear to be hyperthyroid when it's a liver problem. The same can happen if your gut doesn't convert.

When we get sick, I want to see my TSH come up. Why? Because it's increasing metabolism so I can raise my temperature and illicit a proper immune response to whatever thinks it can live in my body. Is this a hypothyroid event? Do I need medication? No. I need my immune system to kick butt and get me well quick.

I could go on for about 10 other pathways, but you get my point. A thyroid patient can also have vitamin D deficiency, iron and/or B12 deficiencies, and many other conditions. This is managed care arrogance. I don't say ignorance, because everyone qualified to order blood tests has passed the test on thyroid cycle.

I need information to make an "educated" guess for my "practice." Otherwise it's an uninformed educated guess, and I'm not able to use the tools I know to run my practice. I'm not bashing any docs here, unless they feel this practice is adequate. In that case, and at some point in their career, they will need a good attorney because they missed something vital to their patient.

Autoimmunity Intestinal Permeability and Nitric Oxide

Intestinal permeability leads to further infections, autoimmunity, chronic fatigue, depression, anxiety, and diabetes type I (especially in children). Also, leads to autism with no familiar history, cardiovascular disease because bacterial endotoxins that trigger cardiovascular inflammatory responses. In turn, an inflammatory bowel reduces the Nitric oxide (NO) pathway. If you recall, this is one of the most important pathways for cardiovascular health. I know we spoke of it earlier, but here is some further explanation regarding autoimmunity.

I will take the time to explain the role of NO in intestinal permeability and the three enzymes for Nitric Oxide Synthase (NOS). This enzyme has three subspecies of NO, neuronal (nNOS), endothelial (eNOS), and inducible (iNOS). eNOS dilates mucosal blood vessels and prevents white blood cell aggregation. It is important to maintain mucosal blood flow and proper digestion. If eNOS is decreased, this results in increased susceptibility of GI track injury. eNOS helps protect against the non-steroidal anti-inflammatory drugs (NSAIDs) because it has antioxidant properties

212

it renders. Furthermore, eNOS helps cardiovascular endothelial tissue recover and regenerate and dissolve endothelial plaque. It dilates blood vessels and enhances blood flow.

nNOS supports neurological function and communication and is neuroprotective. It is located in the nervous tissue and skeletal muscle. Without enough of nNOS, one may be subjected to asthma, restless leg syndrome, and schizophrenia as well as other neurological conditions. nNOS is both in the central and peripheral nervous systems and plays a role in the communication link between the plasma membranes and intracellular communication.

iNOS promotes tissue destruction. It promotes inflammation and autoimmunity and is located in the immune and cardiovascular system via the NF-kappa beta pathway. Its purpose is to be up-regulated inflammation as a defense mechanism. This could be in the case of exposure to pathogens such as bacteria or parasites, but also tumor growth. It is the primary pathway for septic shock and can be a positive feedback mechanism. When unregulated, they self-promote autoimmunity. iNOS is activated by TH 17 pathway and produces harmful free radicals for tissue destruction. This is the pathway in the immunity section that attacks. What is natural that can you use to stop iNOS and the NF-kappa beta pathway? Many are the same as mentioned above. Turmeric, glutathione, and resveratrol. So, is it ok to eat chicken curry and have a glass of red wine, but not the whole bottle of wine? Probably.

When I was undergoing formal education, I saw a special on the Discovery channel where in India they lived in a poor, polluted environment. Where the deceased were often placed and now were floating down the river. They didn't always have access to clean water or quality food. How are they even alive, I wondered? Well, in part, because of a diet high in turmeric and other dietary spices. Turmeric is an anti-inflammatory, anti-oxidant, free radical scavenging, and DNA protective. It is a great start to our management. There's a book called "HEALING SPICES [236]" that has some wonderful concepts and research into ways you can cook and protect your physiology with these natural protectors.

iNOS resides for the most part in the immune system and cardiovascular system. This means once the process has begun, widespread inflammatory processes occur. When it happens, you undergo such as the NF-kappa beta inflammatory cascade. In a very short time, it can go from the gastrointestinal tract, your primary source of immune function, to the cardiovascular, and then your brain.

Not all tests and treatments are perfect, and no one knows everything. You may react perfectly and actually look "cured." Or you could also have all the best treatment, medical and alternative, and have no response. In my office, I don't give up on a patient until I've exhausted all my ideas, good or bad. To this date, I haven't.

Of course, if a tissue doesn't work right, then it's dysfunction decreases the eNOS and nNOS. There is an increase in iNOS that drives NF-kappa beta and increases inflammation. L-Arginine is non-specific and pushes all three pathways. If you have a known autoimmune condition, you may not want to drive it by taking a broad spectrum L-arginine that could be converted to iNOS. Remember, that's the main ingredient in a lot of erectile dysfunction medications and supplements.

One of main causes for autoimmunity is an unmanaged blood sugar handling. Under this particular model, the unmanaged case depletes glutathione in the gastrointestinal tract and liver. Then, your bowels become permeable. The bowel is more susceptible to infections and yeast growth once it becomes permeable. This can also happen under periods of stress and certain medications. Unfortunately, you no longer have the enzymes and bacteria to digest food and it now crosses the gut lumen barrier undigested. The body now has food products it sees as foreign. Now, it must activate an immunological response most of us know as food allergies with the worst culprit being gluten.

We understand that a leaky gut leads to the production of inflammatory hormones in the gut and systemic inflammation. Keep it up and you can have brain fog, poor function, low muscle endurance and strength, decreased energy and fatigue. You wouldn't know anyone like that, would you? Fatigue is hands down the number one reason people go to the doctor. And if most patients with fatigue are autoimmune, shouldn't we be testing it more?

In recap, you need to answer questions like are you sensitive to foods you eat, smells, or chemicals. Do you have current or past antibiotic use? How are your hormones and blood sugar functioning? Any infections, brain trauma, stroke, or a destructive lifestyle? If you are, there's a great deal of possibility that in all likelihood you have a leaky gut. And now you know how that can create autoimmunity.

You need to see a practitioner who will test you for blood sugar, cross-reactants, gluten, inflammation, and Vitamin D for starters and if your condition is gut-related stool testing for pathogens and microbiome. If not, the chances are you will feel better for a while.

But after that, you will be treated again and again and again for rotating infections or symptoms. Or like so many of my patients, bounce from physician to physician until you have a doctor who explains and understands the mechanisms.

In my experience, if we can't get the blood sugar managed and the stress handled, this will continue to degrade. A new stress, an illness, divorce, loss of a loved one, can quickly bring it back because the mechanisms for degradation are already put into place. While this is called a flare, it's our job to understand flares. Also, what triggered them so you can decrease inflammation and slow down destruction.

Here is an example of one autoimmune issue that we see time and time again in our office. The overwhelming majority of patients with autoimmunity are not rheumatoid arthritis, ulcerative colitis, or celiac as the commercials portray. It is instead Hashimoto's thyroiditis. The conventional approach to most thyroid conditions is to monitor a hormone that stimulates the thyroid. This is a thyroid-stimulating hormone or TSH. Then prescribe synthetic, biological, or a combination of thyroid hormones T3 or T4 and monitor TSH to see if you can get it within range, and voila. You're cured.

I have made my career and improved my own health by reading, learning and educating myself about this common autoimmune disease. I don't understand why the vast majority of doctors are not testing for antibodies for the thyroid. Yes, their current treatment protocol won't change. But what they don't tell you is Hashimotos' can go to about anything in the body. It can attack joints, any organ, imbalance hormones, digestion, muscle fatigue, and worse, your brain, and nervous system.

No! I disagree. A good number in the TSH is only about 1/10th of the testing. That's the equivalent of taking your car to a mechanic and saying it shakes, rattles, and rolls. The mechanic nods their head, kicks the tires and says, "You're fine!"

Furthermore, the integration between the nervous and immune systems is very complex. Do you know symptoms of eczema or a rash, headaches, or other symptoms relate to your autoimmunity? Or are they a separate issue? Can you test for it? When a new symptom comes up is that progression or a flare? What triggers the start of a flare? What can you do to stop a flare?

Take a NSAID, steroid, or stop moving. Those are your current options. But that's not your only options. This is why I recommend someone who knows functional medicine and neurology. If you can't get the brain to fire, you won't digest. And if you don't digest, you can't get the products or food to fix the brain, nervous, and immune system. Your body is more delicate and deserving of only looking at one system.

Ask an M.D. in their field what field is most important. To a cardiologist, the heart is the most important. The neurologist says the brain and nervous system. And to the gastroenterologist, the digestive system. I get it. That's their interest. But, without the brain, the heart will cease to beat. Without fuel, it will also cease to beat. Without blood from the heart, you can't digest. And without the nervous system, you don't know where to send blood first to digest. They are all important.

So, if your doctor, alternative or medical, only looks at one part of your body, such as in the example of the TSH, you could have 100 other things festering and screwing up the prescribed medication or therapies. And now you're spinning your wheels. I and my colleagues see this every single day. What I let people know is we have to focus and have a plan on what to focus. Yes, it could be environmental. It could be food, stress, and any physiology issues such as blood supply, hormones, and blood sugar. It could be all of them, or one of them. And that could be today, or five years from now.

How many autoimmune patients have been told they have a lifelong incurable disease? None in my office have until they meet me. That's not always a fun conversation. But this has been swept under the rug by other doctors. So, if you think it's curable, how serious are you on a treatment plan? Or following instructions, thinking, "This couldn't hurt me. I'll be ok." [237] Get tested and find what makes you worse and what makes you better. You'll love yourself more for being in control.

CHAPTER 8

It's All In My Genes, Right? Because It's Genetic, There's Nothing I Can Do About It!

I am a firm believer that you were created to be healthy, and your body wants to be healthy. I believe your body can health itself. Our testing, treatments, and recommendation are tools to support your innate ability to heal. For instance, when you get a paper cut, do you run to the doctor? No. You say ouch, compress, or run under water. The cells around the cut send out cellular messages of cell disruption, the cut, the inflammation and swelling in the area all communicate and your body does what is necessary to fix it. You didn't say, Vain, I need you to heal this cut. This is innate. My job is to help enhance, and in some cases unlock your innate healing, and enhance your body to heal yourself.

I do not want you to be scared of the genetic code that you inherited. I want you to feel like, "Hey, I can put these genes to work for me instead of me thinking or obsessing about what they can do to me." But first, some genetic basics.

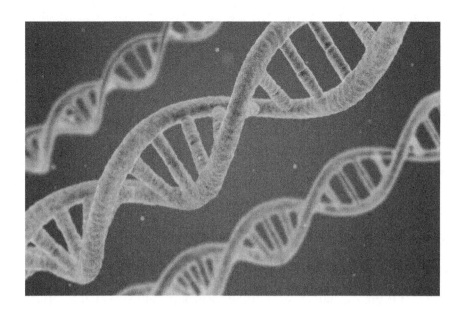

While a genetic program or subsequent programs are not a cure, would you consider doing something to thwart a serious disease for around $3 a day? Most people would agree to this. Here's what we do know. Even if you have all the cards stacked against you from genetics, environment, and lifestyle, that inevitable disease can be slowed down and delayed with the correct nutrition. When it comes to serious diseases such as Alzheimer's, remember, that currently costs $150,000 per year to manage. Three dollars a day for decades is still a good investment, even if it meant starving off for one year without this debilitating disease. Your family is still up $149,000. Adding to Alzheimer's, depression affects 1 in 4 Americans and 25% of women over 40. Ten percent of the population takes mood-altering prescriptions costing $200B a year. [238] [239] [240]

So, what do you do? Methylation is the long-term key. There is nothing in your body that doesn't need to be methylated. Methylation, or methyl groups known in chemistry as CH3, suppresses the expression of viral genes and other harmful stretches of DNA that have been assimilated over time. For instance, if you have one of the well-researched BRCA1 gene of breast cancer, of which there are hundreds known mutations, that is a mutation for you. While you are born with the gene, it is very rare that you are born with breast cancer. Your methyl group hangs over the top of this mutation until another virus, toxin, chemical, stress, dietary insufficiencies or other genetic mutations decrease the production of methyl group. Now, that mutated gene is exposed and has the potential to cause, when turned on, a disease.[241] [242] [243]

The opposite of methylation is called acetylation. So, supplements and foods do this more efficiently. When you have a load of toxins, your body conjugates them with acetyl-CoA. That is also responsible for cholesterol. So, a toxic person makes more cholesterol and they don't recycle it. So, they have higher cholesterol and LDL levels. Again, I must question why the LDL's are elevated. Acetylation pathways are dependent on pantothenic acid, thiamin, and vitamin C. This doesn't mean you will acetylate in taking these. But, if you overdose, it can. The big picture is your body needs to acetylate at times. It opens and repairs. Then, you cover that gene up with a methylation group.

Methylation is dependent on methionine, betaine, ascorbic acid, alpha tocopherol, choline, B6, trimethylglycine, magnesium, B12, and folate. So, when someone has a methylation gene or is told they are not methylating-sufficient. Too often a regiment of B12 or folate is provided. That's so frustrating to me. I continue to repeat myself because this is important. You are more than one gene. Every gene needs adequate methylation and acetylation. Those change over time, through environment and lifestyle.

I will mention sulfation and glucuronidation because they have roles in genetic material. If you eat sulfur-containing foods as suggested in the immune section and take a gall bladder support product, you may manage these without additional help. I bring these up because they have to be addressed in your journey.

Another process many of us are familiar with is glycation. This is where the red blood cells take on sugar. It's the equivalent of caramelizing a pastry or browning something. Most of the time when you are doing this process, you heat sugar. The same thing occurs in your body.

Glycation is tested in your blood with hemoglobin A1C. Most of the time your doctor is monitoring Type I or II diabetes with an A1C test. A side note, Alzheimer's is known as Type III diabetes. Blood sugar imbalances are a big co-factor for glycation. The better your blood sugar, the longer your cells live and repair. [244]

For all of these cycles to work, you must need energy. In your cells, it is the mitochondria where cellular energy (ATP) is made. Without these, or adequate energy, you age and die. Mitochondrial metabolism is the key to aging. In reality you are only as young as their mitochondria. CoQ10 and Ubiquinol feed the mitochondria. Great, take some. Well, you stop making normal amounts of CoQ10 around age 25. It then requires energy to create ubiquinol, the more active form. Adults should take the latter instead of CoQ10. For the most part, adults are taking CoQ10 for energy. But you need ubiquinol that requires energy to convert. It's frustrating to take a product that requires energy when you're taking a product for energy. For longevity and methylation, you need blood to transport nutrients. More importantly, you need that to get blood to your brain. It needs to methylate, detoxify, repair, and be fed too.[245]

Loss of methylation has the capability to impact three major disease factors, infection, toxicity, and stress. Methylation genetic mutations can lead to chronic disease, increased environmental toxin burden, and have secondary effects on genetic expression. It can also lead to emotional instability. This occurs because you don't make neurotransmitters efficient without methylation.[246]

The main function of methylation is to turn genes on and off. It also detoxifies and builds and metabolizes neurotransmitters, such as norepinephrine, epinephrine (adrenalin) serotonin, dopamine, and melatonin. Methylation also processes hormones such as estrogen, insulin, and cortisol. It builds the immune cells especially T-cells and natural killer cells.

Going further as you age, you need additional DNA synthesis and repair, production of energy such as CoQ10 and ATP. Also, you need the production of myelin covering the nerves, and maintaining cell membranes. The discrepancy from one person to another on how efficient their methylation cycle run determines how fast we age. As you can see, most diseases and conditions have one or more of these impairments that require methylation.

There are several known factors that disrupt methylation:

-Lack of nutrients such as zinc, B2, magnesium, B6, B12, folate

-Medications (antacids, methotrexate, metformin, nitrous oxide deplete methyl groups as do many others)

-Specific nutrient depleting dietary intake of these nutrients including the inflammatory foods from above

-Environmental toxicity, heavy metals, chemicals, pesticides, herbicides, fungicides

-Genetic mutations that you inherited

-Stress can also influence methylation. Over exertions via physical, chemical, mental, emotional are all forms of stress. It doesn't matter where the stress is from, as far as your body is concerned, it all counts.[247 248 249 250 251]

The more methylated a gene is, the less active it is. Methylation can be tested through blood tests. B12, folic acid, homocysteine, liver enzymes, red blood cell size, and antibodies can give an idea what methylation is occurring. You can run more precise genetic testing through blood, mouth swab, and saliva. Methylation is involved in almost every biochemical reaction, and occurs billions of times every second in our cells. It manages or contributes to a wide range of crucial body functions. That's why figuring out where the methylation cycle can better perform is a big deal. When looking at methylation, you can't look only at blood or genes. You have to compare them both. Then advise or test what allows improvement and/or reduces symptoms. Please don't stop there. This is a health journey. Continue to test blood and urine because it will tell you what is working, what needs additional support, and what is now needing help.

Below is a basic list of what methylation does for you:

Detoxification

-Immune function

-Maintaining DNA and DNA repair and turning genes off and on

-Energy production

-Mood balancing through balancing of neurotransmitters

-Controlling inflammation

-Maintaining integrity of cell membranes

-Processes hormones

-Keeps the nervous system conducting with efficiency

With any health condition, the question to ask is: Why and how did this happen? In the past, people believed that all health conditions sprang from one cause, like a bug or toxin. But now the latest science reveals that many factors acting together can produce illness. That's why to understand complex health problems, we must identify the multiple contributing factors. A combination of genetic weaknesses, metal toxicities, infections, and other factors can lead to negative events. If your doctor looks at these, you should have a customized step-by-step process that helps you address all factors in an individualized treatment plan.[252] [253] [254]

Why do we run these genetic tests? If you've ever been tested for the flu or any other disease or condition, you want to be negative. Positive (+) means something isn't working. Like HIV positive. That is the same in the case of genes. Positive Positive (++ or +-) this means you are positive for a genetic mutation. It does not mean it is no longer functioning. When you have a ++ gene, that gene functions, but at best around 30 percent. When you have a +- gene, that gene functions too. But at best, 70%. This is why it takes time for most diseases to occur. Genes code for amino acids, the building blocks for proteins. These make enzymes, neurotransmitters, antibodies and most forms of physiology responsible for life.[255] [256] [257]

This leads me to a very important point. Many people have shelled out thousands of dollars on genetic testing. But their doctor didn't test for digestion or question their dietary intake. Without adequate protein, you cease efficient function. Over time you gain a myriad of symptoms and conditions. Add some time and you gain a diagnosis. The purpose of a genetic test is to evaluate the major genes that support the major functions of life. If necessary, recommend nutritional options that have been researched to support these genes. But, and a big one, if you can't digest or break down recommended foods or supplements, your expectation should be very low. I see this as a fundamental flaw in our healthcare system, regardless of the doctor. You must digest so your body can take those nutrients and repair them.

The Human Genome Project is an international scientific research project. Its goal is to determine the sequence of chemical base pairs which make up human DNA, then identify and map all of the genes of the human genome from both a physical and functional standpoint. The genome was mapped a decade ago and further research has been made on specific genes. This group has discovered many mutations, inheritance, and disease pathways and opened the door to additional research.[258]

What are single nucleotide polymorphisms (SNPs)?

These are single nucleotide polymorphisms, often called SNPs (pronounced "snips"). These are the most common type of genetic variation among people. Each SNP represents a difference in a single DNA building block, called a nucleotide. Pieces of the nucleotide are denoted as A, T, G, and C. Everything your body produces is in response to a series of these four nucleotides. A SNP may replace the nucleotide cytosine (C) with the nucleotide thymine (T) in a certain stretch of DNA. SNPs occur throughout a person's DNA, and this is normal variation. In fact, they occur once in every 300 nucleotides on average, which means there are roughly 10 million SNPs in the human genome. More common, these variations, also called mutations, are found in the DNA between genes. They can act as biological markers. These markers help scientists locate genes that are associated with disease.

When SNPs occur within a gene or in a regulatory region near a gene, they may play a more direct role in disease by affecting the gene's function. Often a SNP is caused by exposure to environmental changes, toxins, viruses, and other pathogens, chemicals, and lack of nutrients consumed. That SNP could have been from your father being exposed to agent orange in Vietnam, or a great-grandparent being exposed to the toxins of the industrial revolution. Or it could have been our forefathers going through periods of starvation. Now you have the mutation.

While most SNPs have no effect on health or development, some of these genetic differences have proven to be very important in the study of human health. Researchers have found SNPs that may help predict an individual's response to certain drugs, susceptibility to environmental factors such as toxins, and the risk of developing particular diseases. SNPs can also be used to track the inheritance of disease genes within families. Future studies will work to identify SNPs associated with complex diseases such as heart disease, diabetes, and cancer, and are critical for individual and specialized treatments.

Mutations create genetic diversity, which keeps populations healthy. (Survival of the fittest). Keep in mind, many mutations have no effect at all. These are called silent mutations. But when you first see a genetic report and observe all the mutations you have, it can be daunting.

A person could have more than 1 million snips, but only about 40,000 snips are known to alter genetic function. Many of my patients have sent away for the genetic tests, and companies come back stating they needed to take massive amounts of nutrition to support all of these genes. Now they've been recommended to spend thousands of dollars a month in nutrition that makes compliance very hard to follow. Not to mention it will make you broke. How can one follow recommendations that doesn't allow input for food or changes in your environment? I see a lot of doctors who don't offer more than one genetic report. When you're looking at genes, you need to communicate with yourself, or in my case, your client, on what affects their genes.

Introduction to Epigenetics

Often, the genes tested in your genome are not specific for a pathological disease. These would include BRCA1, BRCA2, and ER2 genes when evaluating breast cancer, for example. However, in many of those cases and other major diseases they have a defunct vitamin D receptor (VDR). Also, lessened detoxification pathways (MTHFR, MTR, MTRR, SUOX, CBS,) and many others that we test. Should you have a family history of those diseases, it is still recommended to have specific genetic testing, regardless of the outcome of this program.[259] [260]

Although additional mutations can occur at any time during our lifetime, you are born with many mutations and you will have them throughout your life. These inherited mutations have been passed down to us from previous generations (our parents and grandparents) and may be passed to future generations (our children). This provides an explanation about why certain traits or diseases run in the family. Although we cannot change our genetic code, we can change how our genes are expressed. Research has revealed that our gene expression is not determined by only hereditary factors. But it is also influenced by our diet, nutritional status, toxic load, and environmental influences, or stressors. This phenomenon has been termed "epigenetics."

Researchers in the growing field of epigenetics have demonstrated that certain genes can be over- or under-expressed with certain disease processes. Ongoing research hopes that by understanding how these genes are regulated and what is influencing them, we may be able to change their expression. Using epigenetic concepts along with a good understanding of the methylation cycle, researchers have begun to make recommendations to optimize genetic expression and help to restore health.

Recent progress in the understanding of nutritional influences on epigenetics suggests that nutrients that are part of methyl-group metabolism. In short, nutrition does influence your epigenetics. [261] [262]

Of course, you could have an APO-E4 with an MTHFR, or a lot of brain trauma and toxins, that may be a more difficult case. But below are things you have complete control over.[263] [264] [265]

Epigenetic Support, Regardless Of Your Inheritance

It will always be good to buy organic and use healthy and what's considered "green" products. Regardless of what you do, your body still has to deal with many toxins, even those that come from natural organic foods. Each day you are eating three to four pounds a food and breathing in several thousand liters of air. That alone is a lot of detoxification that your body must go through on a daily basis.

Understanding how life influences their genes, positive or negative, can be beneficial to you. Too many doctors focus on one gene known as the MTHFR. I want you to know that you are more than one gene with a potential for thousands of snips. It is preposterous to focus on one SNP.

Most of the reports we get are somewhat in this format below. Red means you have two out of two mutations, yellow is one of two mutations, and white or sometimes green is no mutations. Keep in mind, you could have no mutations for the lung but work in a coal mine, smoke three packs a day, and sleep in the mud and you will probably still have lung issues. Genetics are important, but they're not everything.

Gene	RS	Risk Allele	Your Genotype		Category	Related Factors
VDR	rs12717991	T	TT	++	Immune/Mineral Balance	T Cells , Vitamin D , Infections (Bacteria, virus etc.), Insulin, L. Dopa, Lactose, Phenylalanine, Tryptophan, Tyrosine
VDR	rs886441	G	AA	--	Immune/Mineral Balance	T Cells , Vitamin D , Infections (Bacteria, virus etc.), Insulin, L. Dopa, Lactose, Phenylalanine, Tryptophan, Tyrosine
VDR	rs2189480	T	TT	++	Immune/Mineral Balance	T Cells , Vitamin D , Infections (Bacteria, virus etc.), Insulin, L. Dopa, Lactose, Phenylalanine, Tryptophan, Tyrosine
VDR	rs3782905	C	GG	--	Immune/Mineral Balance	T Cells , Vitamin D , Infections (Bacteria, virus etc.), Insulin, L. Dopa, Lactose, Phenylalanine, Tryptophan, Tyrosine
VDR	rs2238136	T	CT	-+	Immune/Mineral Balance	T Cells , Vitamin D , Infections (Bacteria, virus etc.), Insulin, L. Dopa, Lactose, Phenylalanine, Tryptophan, Tyrosine
VDR (BSM)	rs1544410	T	CC	--	Immune/Mineral Balance	T Cells , Vitamin D , Infections (Bacteria, virus etc.), Insulin, L. Dopa, Lactose, Phenylalanine, Tryptophan, Tyrosine
VDR (Taq)	rs731236	A	AA	++	Immune/Mineral Balance	T Cells , Vitamin D , Infections (Bacteria, virus etc.), Insulin, L. Dopa, Lactose, Phenylalanine, Tryptophan, Tyrosine
MTHFR A1298C	rs1801131	G	GG	++	Methylation	Folic Acid
MTHFR C677T	rs1801133	A	GG	--	Methylation	Folic Acid

We need to look at the big picture and it is very rarely one single SNP. In other words, find the reason that somebody's having health issues. Your body is complex. So, taking one supplement for one SNP isn't enough.

In our office, a lot of new soon-to-be-mothers are concerned about their genetic outcome. Or they're wanting to get pregnant and they are requesting a lot of clarification. I'm asked, What should I take? If you didn't know, most of your prenatals aren't that great. It's more than taking folate. If you didn't know, the neural tube defects and the congenital heart issues are not from a lack of folic acid, but instead a problem in the methylation process which has multiple genes mutated. Most doctors are not aware of this. But if you're wanting to get pregnant, we want both partners methylating with efficiency. Here is where it gets even more confusing and downright frustrating from my perspective. If you don't have an advanced degree in nutrition or biochemistry, then the word folate versus the word folate acid doesn't sound a lot different. The problem is that folic acid stops methylation! Many foods are enriched or enhanced with methylation stopping folate acid. What a pregnant woman needs is folate—they're completely different. [266] [267] [268]

Of the genetic outcome, there are other things that are a detriment to methylation and slow it down. These are alcohol, medications, heavy metals, infections, free radicals, and any sources of inflammation regardless of where they come from.

You need to be able to digest. And, you need to be able to digest protein. For vegetarians and vegans, it really doesn't matter what your genetic code is because your brain and your nervous system need choline. And while there are some in vegetables, it's not enough to support human methylation. They must supplement. And sometimes, supplementation isn't enough. I recommend all vegans and vegetarians get blood tests every 90 days. You don't need a full panel. At the minimum, blood tests for blood sugar, thyroid, and protein absorption. Waiting longer than that can require much more of an effort to correct.

If you have genetic testing combined with blood tests, I will suggest learning about them for few weeks after you've had your results for both. Then, run events through your life thinking about choices and events from the past that may have allowed expression. Then, look towards the future. Ask yourself questions. Will this food, supplement, exercise or other activity have a positive or negative effect on my genes? Like the immune system, you need sleep, hydration, proper exercise, stress relief, and nutrients. Will it help you gain the health you deserve, or make you worse?

Keep in mind life happens. Don't linger on what happened, no guilt, or self-flogging. Start your health with your next opportunity, bite, or meal. Get up in the morning and think, "What do I need to eat to be successful today?" That could change your life one day at a time. Is it a Saturday, and you're doing yard work? Do you have a presentation at work or school, or are you running a marathon? You can see life can throw changes in what you need and how you need to prepare yourself.

Make sure your home has clean water with a water filter that does more than filtering chlorine. Regarding chlorine, a shower filter is also important to keep methylation blockers from getting on your skin. There is a link to a few filters and other household aides in the reference section at the end of this book.

Avoid commercial house cleaners as they are often toxic. Clean your air ducts and have a maintenance schedule for your filters and HVAC. Maintenance will save your health care dollars! That also goes for sink traps and drain pipes where mold can grow and some other nasty stuff. If you don't know how or don't want to, there are handymen available on safe background check sites who can run these on a schedule. We even purchased a gas detector to make sure there aren't any simple leaks as gas can lead to headaches, nausea, dizziness, and all kinds of issues where the house isn't going to blow up. That's great, but you still feel awful. Also, other cleaning materials, cosmetics, soaps, and lotions can also be genetic disruptors. Again, a link to alternatives in the reference section. [269]

Not all of this is as easy to implement. I get it. I've been there before and at times find new triggers. Working with a coach is important. If you don't live in Dallas and don't want to travel or need someone local, here are some tips. Look into references for someone with multiple disciplines. Only having functional medicine, functional neurology, or nutritional/genetic education isn't enough. What is their schedule? I don't know how to see someone new in under an hour. I spend 3-4 hours reading all their material. I also don't know how to explain labs in 15 minutes or less. You have to know where you're going so you're not repeating your health challenges. You need it all. You deserve it all. Those practitioners do exist.

CHAPTER 9

Food Sensitivities (Allergies) and What To Eat For Your Health

For the most part, we have a Standard American Diet, SAD for short. We are 35th in world health, yet for decades, we have been first in spending. That's not the number we should be focused on. Spending is not prevention. So, I've decided to write down a few highlights to get everyone started. Because we live in a toxic world, 350 different pesticides, 75,000 chemicals utilized in industry, new carpets, xenohormones, and on and on. It's obvious we can't avoid being exposed. I like my carpet where I watch football games. However, we can take efforts by being responsible for our environments and what goes into and on our bodies. I will go into everyday toxins in the next chapter because it does affect digestion. DIE-T is a four-letter word that doesn't work. Lifestyle modification works. I promise you that you can do anything if you're big enough. You may have to modify, change, adapt, and integrate any plan. But you can do it.

Food allergies and sensitivities have become much more common in today's world. They are very complex and vastly overlooked when a health problem arises. The most common way to test for food allergies is with a blood test followed by an elimination diet. Certain questionable allergic foods are eliminated from the diet for 3-9 months. Then they are reintroduced. This is easier said than done.

Many people are allergic to their favorite foods and they crave them because that cannot absorb them. Often allergies are created by structural disturbances and become neurological. Some food allergies are due to food being introduced in infancy instead of one at a time. As an infant, or if you are introducing food to a small child coming off of breastfeeding or formula, one should introduce 1-3 foods a week separate from other foods.

The microbiome of your child and of you consists of all the cells that are not human in nature. This means in the womb and during natural birth. A child's microbiome is inhibited by cesarean. The microbiome is 50-55% of your body weight from cells that are symbiotic with us. It is made of bacteria, yeast, fungi, and parasites. Gains in strength and tolerance are noted in infants when given foods one at a time to identify, metabolize, and dampen inflammation. When we have patients with a lot of microbiome issues, we start them with a very diverse shake to help decrease the inflammation. The plan is so they can absorb the food and nutrition that we are suggesting for their case. It's also for diversity, which will help their microbiome. We combine this shake with an in-home pulse test for subtle food sensitivities. Remember, this is not those who are anaphylactic or are known to have trips to the ER for food allergies. Don't test them that way. Seek medical advice about dangerous or anaphylactic allergies.

To run an in-home food allergy test, select suspected foods or a food group and avoid them for three weeks. Read all labels. You may be surprised that a particular food, such as gluten or MSG, is in so many foods. Even a small amount like a bite can trigger a negative allergic response. These are not full borne anaphylaxis allergies. That is a different antibody and very severe. They are food allergies causing inflammation and decreased function. Avoidance allows the body to clear the immune properties. When you begin to reintroduce a suspected food or foods, do it one food at a time. Eat that food throughout the day along with non-allergic foods, paying attention to any reactions. This could be headaches, dizziness, nausea, or other symptoms you've had that have gone away or decreased during the three-week period. If you have a reaction, you need to avoid it for 60-90 days. Wait three days before reintroducing the next food if you have more than one sensitivity or questioned food.

The most common are wheat, gluten, milk, peanuts, corn, and milk. Soy, sugar, citrus, shellfish, coffee, and food additives are second. Look for replacement foods before beginning or you may feel starved, even though you're not. Replacements can help you cope with the loss of something once savored.

How can you tell if anything is good or bad? Again, check your body. If you eat a food and your pulse says 60 beats per minute, and after eating a possibly problematic food the pulse goes up more than 10 beats per minute, you will want to remove the food from the diet for 90 days because this is a positive pulse test. If in 90 days it tests okay with your pulse, you may eat it in rotation, but not daily. This is how you most likely had the problem to begin with.

If you're home and you have 10 weeks to simplify and decide what is inflammatory or not, here are a few things to review in terms of food. You'll want to observe to see if it'll affect your mood, energy, and brain through elimination. When you eliminate the foods and you add them back, you'll find out if they're inflammatory. Most of the time you get an inflammatory response. A symptom, a headache, fatigue or pain. Remember, there are a lot of variables for a diet ,whether that is blood type, lifestyle, or common allergies.

If you're not doing it already, limit gluten, dairy, sugar, soy, eggs, corn, nightshade vegetables, alcohol, and refined foods. This is when you should start. I know it sounds like a lot. You can eat as many dark, leafy green vegetables, and other vegetables, and fruit in the beginning. You can have nuts and seeds and healthy sources of animal protein, which means they are free range grass and grass-fed, antibiotic free. If this doesn't work, we start taking some of these away when you are autoimmune or have severe digestive issues.

If you are a sugar addict, sticking this out for three weeks will help with your sugar cravings. You might also find that symptoms such as bloating, sinus congestion, and excess gas also reduce or go away. Introduce one of these inflammatory foods once you've passed your two or three weeks or none. Observe symptoms, and in three days, introduce another. So, let's say you ate corn on the 15th day, and all of a sudden you bloat or swell and you haven't been doing that for a little bit. That's a great indicator that corn is a problem. You'll need to wait three days or more until the swelling is gone before you introduce another food.

Charting your foods is recommended so you know what is good and what isn't and when you can eat them again, if ever. If a method has failed, a food allergy sensitivity test can be ordered through your doctor or on our website. However, this is buyer beware regarding food sensitivity testing. Most food sensitivity companies test only raw food. My question is, how many people eat raw beef, chicken ,or fish? Not many. There's a difference between how your body reacts or has the ability to react to raw or cooked food. If and when you are tested, you need both of these tested.

Furthermore, one may not be allergic in food allergy testing to wheat, tomato, or cheese individually. But combine them together in something called a pizza, it changes the expression of the proteins. And yes, one can indeed be allergic to pizza and not the individual ingredients. Frustrating, yes. But a doctor who understands this can help you get there. The gold standard for any food allergy testing is Elisa blood serum testing. Skin scratch and cytotoxic testing are hard to reproduce, and in my humble opinion, a waste of good money.

If you didn't hear me before, a strong word of caution. Do not self-test any severe allergic foods! This rotation does not work for these types of allergies as it is a completely different mechanism and you are putting yourself in harm's way.

Carbohydrates – A Sugar Providing Temporary Energy. But When Refined it Starves Life

Again, refined carbohydrates cause problems because they promote illness. By definition, refined carbohydrates are items such as sucrose, glucose, dextrose, high-fructose corn sugar, corn syrup, and other additives in our foods. Natural sugar in fruit and other whole foods do not have refined sugar, although not everyone can tolerate even healthy grains or sugar. In a typical American diet, over 20% of our calories come from refined sugar, or 41 teaspoons of sugar a day! [270] [271]A 12 oz soft drink contains more than eight teaspoons of sugar. Consider the typical person who drinks more than one soda per day. Adding pies, cookies, candies, pastries, cereals, applesauce, and other sweetened foods to our daily intake and 41 teaspoons a day. Your body has to offset, buffer, and detoxify with this bombardment of carbohydrates.

Sugar is a major contributor of fatigue, depression, anxiety, insomnia, PMS, headaches, joint pains, and abdominal complaints. It causes dysglycemia, or an imbalance of blood sugar. High or low, unstabilized blood sugar is detrimental to health and is a causative factor in many disease states. The negative effects suffered from sugar manifests because of its rapid absorption into the bloodstream. It is inefficient energy. This is why you want to run energy from fat. Not only is fat nine calories per vs sugar and protein that are four, but there's more energy in fat. Sugar gets used quickly and has you wanting more. Burning protein takes energy to convert to sugar. This is how you lose more weight on a protein diet compared to a sugar diet even though they have the same caloric amount. The quick uptake of sugar is not an efficient process. Because of this, it requires an excess insulin to be released. An increase in insulin tends to push blood sugar down, but it can't be produced at an elevated level for eternity.

Insulin is a hormone produced in the pancreas. Hormones of any type are regulated by the liver. Raising one hormone decreases others because they need the same building blocks to be produced. Many other enzymatic processes can be reduced or hindered. To keep one from going into a diabetic coma under the influence of so many carbohydrates, the adrenals release epinephrine to vasodilate. This expands the arteries and gets the sugar to the tissue ASAP. Eating too much sugar causes wide swings in blood sugar and elevated levels of regulatory hormones. Over time, the adrenals are forced to put out excess cortisol that binds to the insulin, causing insulin resistance. Add a few more high blood sugar incidences over a few months, and the red blood cells (RBC's) become crystallized with sugar known as hemoglobin A1C. The RBC's bound to sugar then scratch the inside of the arteries and vascular system, giving the platelets an area to bind to (adhere). Along comes cholesterol to cover up the platelet aggregation, and now you have plaque.

For repair, plaque is good, as long as it can be removed right after the healing is completed. But that's not in most Americans' arteries. They are oxidizing and promoting more plaque formation. Once cholesterol plaque formation is oxidized due to lack of oxygen (limited movement), and you continue free radicals exposure from unhealthy lifestyles, stress, and more bad food choices, then the cholesterol becomes more sticky and binds more platelets and cholesterol. The bigger the clog, the more there is a decrease in blood flow. This is why diabetics are at a much higher risk for cardiovascular incidents such as stroke, heart attack, and pulmonary embolism. And this is why these events are on their death certificate and not diabetes.

So, what do we do? Is this an aspirin deficiency or perhaps a cholesterol toxicity as promoted in our media advertisements? Considering the mechanisms previously mentioned, I do not agree! It's a sugar problem. And continued usage leads to many pathological conditions including diabetes, cardiovascular disease, erectile dysfunction, migraines, decreased immunity, and toxic conditions. These physiological changes are what in the beginning contribute to hypoglycemia, and low blood sugar.

While other issues are too much adrenaline, eating too much sugar while you're still at a decent level of health will over time become hyperglycemia, high blood sugar, and then metabolic syndrome, syndrome X, insulin resistance, and Type II diabetes. You may have heard of these. When type II diabetics are not regulated, you can go from non-insulin dependent to insulin dependent. This is where you must take insulin just as a Type 1 diabetic.

A good idea is to find balance when consuming sugar. Many Americans do reach for a salad, but with a boatload of dressing that's full of trans-unsaturated fats and sugar, and lose the benefit. Or they reach for the number one vegetable consumed in the United States. If you didn't know, potatoes are a carbohydrate, as are many vegetables. No, I didn't say you get a pass from vegetables, just those that are high is starch. A synonym for sugar is starch. Foods with sugar or starch, or have a high glycemic index, meaning how fast the vegetable sugars get into your body.

Here's a fun fact. Diabetes growth in the U.S. is directly proportional to cola sales. The average U.S. citizen eats 160 pounds of sugar in one year and drinks 60 gallons of pop. How many do you consume? How does that affect you? How does that affect your genetic expression and future generations? [272]

A Glass of Wine, a Beer, a Cocktail? No Harm, Right?

Alcohol—when is it ok? Alcohol will damage the liver as well as destroy the brain. Alcohol kills brain cells that are important in communicating function to your body. Other organs are also implicated with its consumption such as the gastrointestinal tract and the pancreas. Alcohol is a sugar by nature and causes an acidic imbalance. This impairs the immune system and allows processes such as yeast, bacteria, virus, mold, fungus, parasites, and unfortunately cancer, to go unnoticed. Those who are carbohydrate intolerant suffer the same effects as a full-blown alcoholic, even with small amounts of alcohol consumption. Their body can at times convert sugar to alcohol. Or the intestines have the wrong bacteria and convert carbohydrates to alcohol. That's rough.

Drinking alcohol can aggravate other conditions such as gout, psoriasis (an autoimmune skin condition), hormone imbalance and detoxification ability. Although cardiovascular disease is decreased with populations who drink moderate amounts of red wine, this is due to the substance known as resveratrol. There are other avenues to have the benefit of wine without the risk of alcohol. Other than antiseptic implications, there doesn't seem to be a clear-cut beneficial health reason to consume.

Fats

Let's talk about fats. There are good fats, bad fats, and meh fats. Your body has a process to utilize them. There was a movement in the late 80's and early 90's to get this fat out of our food. Many food manufacturers, under the guise that fat causes heart disease, pulled fats out in lieu of some junk research and inserted sugar. It was mainly replaced with high fructose corn syrup instead. Well, sugar turns to fat and creates metabolic demands that push you towards diabetes, permeable intestines, autoimmunity, and many other disease states. So, you can pull the fat out of the food product and you can still get fat and sick eating them. That sucks! Move forward three decades, and those foods made of sugar, salt, and fat are still dominating the vending machines.

When it comes to fat, you need to know what is good and what is bad. Bad is trans or trans-unsaturated also known as hydrogenated fat. Margarine is an example of what this is. While these are edible, they increase the risk of coronary artery disease and lower the good cholesterol, HDL. This increases systemic inflammation. I'm sure you already know the number one veggie eaten in the U.S. is french fries.

Here's a fun fact for those fries you may be thinking about right now. Each serving, and many current portions are beyond a serving. Think a small size in a paper sack from the biggest fast-food chain as an actual serving size. Each serving contains five grams of trans fats. Ok, what does that mean? It means it takes approximately one entire year for that amount to leave your body. That means your blood sugar, insulin, detoxification, antioxidant, and other systems are compromised. And, for a long period of time. Even the majority of all the cells in your body will be replaced before the trans-fat has been eliminated! Even longer if you get the "normal" serving size.

Good fats are produced from vegetables, fish oils, eggs, and free-range, grass-fed animal meat. I hear often, "Isn't there studies that eggs are full of fat that are both good and bad for you? And what about fish oils being both good and bad for you?"

This is where we get to understand the difference between omegas. You need 3, 6, 9, with the majority being 3. Omega 9 is a small player and the main ones are omegas 3 and 6. There is a healthy ratio between 3 and 6 that needs to be 1:4 or less. Our Neanderthal ancestors were closer to 1:1 and didn't show signs of chronic disease. The average American is 25:1 or more and why we exhibit more disease states. Healthy omega 3 fats are ALA (flax), DHA, and EPA found in marine sources (salmon, trout, herring, krill).

They're in free range, antibiotic-free, grass-fed meats; wild-caught fish; and free-range, antibiotic-free, cage free eggs.

Omega 3 stops inflammation by inhibiting inflammatory pathways. Unhealthy omega-6 fats are fried foods (saturated and trans fats), junk food, dairy, soy, and corn. They do not stop the inflammatory process, but instead promote it. So, when you are in pain, bloating or inflamed you are creating more of a problem eating these things.[273]

The studies on fish oils or eggs that state these foods are bad for you are because those animals were fed grains or soy that are rich in omega 6. When you eat omega 6 food, you will become inflamed, and increase the disease-promoting process.[274]

Choosing to eat fewer fats is also detrimental. Low-fat diets lead to clinical depression, mood swings, tremors, brain fog, fatigue, and many other neurological findings. This is because each nerve cell is coated with healthy fats to increase the neurological transmission of signals. The coating of a nerve cell is called the myelin sheath. The old adage "you are what you eat" should also include "you are what your food eats and grows."

Concerning fats, many Americans take cholesterol-lowering drugs because they are still under the impression that all fat is bad. There are actually good and bad fats. Many of these drugs to treat high cholesterol fall into a class known as statin drugs. What consumers don't know is there is no change in death rates from heart disease, myocardial infarction, or stroke using these medications. [275] [276]. Then, may I ask, what are you taking them for?

Cholesterol is needed in all cells for life. If there is an issue, genetic snips for APO-E and MTHFR from our genetic chapter should be evaluated. Or if one has been tested for cholesterol size, risk, arterial inflammation, and other factors, then I don't see a reason to bring in medications. Those patients are high risk and should consider medical help. In fact, there are several blood tests that I prefer and understand. They are more superior to cholesterol when understanding cardiovascular risk. Research has shown homocysteine is more indicative than cholesterol as is C-Reactive Protein (CRP). Cholesterol has a cycle. It is necessary for hormones, the brain, the immune system, and when you have inflammation, LDL (bad cholesterol) goes to the site of inflammation. It is recycled back by HDL. Also, LDL is required in every cell of your body, so why are you getting rid of it? Was God, nature, or whatever created you wrong with the cholesterol thing? Research is significant that cardiovascular disease is reversible if one changes their diet to anti-inflammatory. Oh, yeah—those essential fatty acids are great to reduce cholesterol numbers.

Microwave

What if I'm in a hurry, will it be hurt if I eat out, junk food, what if I microwave it? All questions I hear in my office, and for the most part it's situational. What is a microwave and what does it do to your food? Is it a good starting point? I encourage you to look up Kirlian photography with microwaves and apples and Kirlian photography with water. Microwave is radiation so you are radiating your food. Cells don't stay healthy with radiation.[277]

Microwaves work by causing water friction, and the friction heats up your food, and kills good nutrients. Many vitamins and minerals are only water soluble, and when radiated, they become useless. Only Vitamins A, D , E, K, fat, and oils (empty calories) are preserved through microwaving. So, are you gaining nutritional value? Not unless it's a fat, and if it's a bad fat, it's inflammatory. That's how fast food can contain calories but not have much nutritional value.

Here are some simple yet practical rules and facts to live by:

•Things to avoid: commercial fruits and veggies, processed meats

•Limit allergens: milk, chocolate, soy, wheat, peanut, and the foods above. They increase fatigue, bloating, depression, brain fog, decrease performance and add to inflammation and pain.

•Reduce/Remove junk food and bad carbs from the diet, eating a variety of healthful, nutrient-rich foods.

•If the list of ingredients is not on the package, it may not healthy

•Choose an alkaline diet. No disease or pathogenic organism has been shown to live in an alkaline diet. Acidic diets are rich in white sugar, refined foods and dairy.

•Eat foods that rot or spoil, but do it before it does, which means you should eat foods as close to nature as possible or how it was 100 years ago. This food has life, and bugs know what will sustain life. Bugs are not altered or influenced by the media, they can't read. Insects are only concerned with what will sustain life. If it won't sustain their life, it won't sustain yours. Good bread grows mold in one week as an example. Please don't think most bread is good for you.

•Eat as much color as possible. Phytochemistry, nutrients from plants. Color protects versus aging, degeneration, and DNA mutation. The microbiome mash is rich in biodiversity.

•Shop around the edge of the shopping center. All the good stuff is here. All the inflammatory and disease-promoting foods are in the middle, all boxed and preserved for your enjoyment.

•Canned is worse but only if necessary, frozen is better, and fresh and organic best. We have to eat. Sometimes for our family and budget, we have to get what we can and make the best choices we can with our individual situations.

•Cage-free chicken eggs with no hormones, omega-3 fatty acids, and no antibiotics are best. A cage-free chicken eats different a diet of bugs and grass. You need to make sure they don't get grains as a supplement to their diet. Most companies have a website, and the ones I like have stories about their chickens.

•Eat three meals with snacks between. Aim for an appropriate amount of carbohydrate for each meal and snack according to your level of health and activity. Balance protein, essential fats, non-processed foods. This is different if you are on an intermittent fasting plan. I recommend only 16 hours at the max and 10-12 as the minimum between meals if you are on this.

•Get adequate rest and appropriate exercise. This helps you digest and have a reasonable yet not overactive desire for food.

•What if you eat fried foods with trans fats? Remember, they block pain reducers and increase inflammation. Try to consume or supplement with good fats as soon as possible, but don't make a habit of consuming these inflammatory foods.

•Most diseases can be prevented or reversed with what you eat.

•Your body is brilliant at adapting to prevent failures, but not without a cost. One must find and eliminate the influences that cause these negative influences on your health.

Specific Food Programs

There are some you know, and some may be new to you. Let's start with physiology. There is a difference between hunger and cravings. If you have cravings, you're missing nutrients. It's hard to not turn your brain off when you are joshing for something. Do your best to get it out of your head. Eat something healthy, asking yourself if you need to eat it or do you want to eat it. Honesty goes a long way here as we can justify just about anything in our own minds.

FODMAPS

For those who have bad intestinal issues or struggle with irritable or inflammatory bowels, you have an autoimmune bowel. You may consider the FODMAPs for a few months. The term 'FODMAP' is an acronym for Fermentable Oligo-, Di-, Mono-saccharides, and Polyols. In short, they are fermentable carbohydrates found in many of the foods we often eat. If you are on FODMAPs or considering it, you should consider working with a professional. Also get tested for permeable membrane and bowel infections so you know how to help yourself.

Autoimmune Paleo

Many of our autoimmune patients are on the autoimmune Paleo diet (AIP) which looks exactly like elimination without nuts. The goal is to restore your microbiome. You do this by eating as much variety as possible. If your symptoms are going from an 8/10 and to a 5/10 or lower, you know that this is working. But you also know this doesn't happen overnight.[278] [279] [280]

Ketogenic

The ketogenic diet has been very successful with those who have brain disorders such as epilepsy or seizures. There's a brain modulator when you're in ketogenesis called beta hydroxybutyrate made in the liver. While in keto, this helps create energy in the brain. It doesn't matter how you get there, whether it's plant-based protein or animal-based protein. Beta hydroxybutyrate affects the immune system and helps support certain regions of the brain and genetic expression of BDNF. A proper ketogenic diet consists of a lot of fibers. Particularly green-leaf vegetables. The ones that have the highest amount of fiber are best such as swiss chard, bok choy, spinach, kale, and arugula with some sort of protein combined with it. In a perfect keto program, you cycle through four weeks with measurements. You still need blood tests before and after with measurements of urine every three to seven days to make sure that you are in ketosis. For menopausal women who started gaining weight with menopause, or women gaining fat on the back of their arms which is very hard lose, the term for this is estrogen dominance. Keto is beneficial to reducing estrogen dominance, and it supports female physiology.

The caveats and warnings come before going on a keto diet. You need to make sure that you can digest food first, especially fat, because that's been your macronutrient. So, if you don't digest fat or have a gallbladder issue, your stool floats. If you have low vitamin D or low cholesterol, the ketogenic diet isn't going to work very well for you. And if you still want to, you need to fix fat digestion first.

Intermittent Fasting

You can start intermittent fasting or consider it as an option as long as you are not hypoglycemic. With intermittent fasting you need to be fasting for at least 12 hours minimum with 16 hours being the max. With intermittent fasting, as the day goes on, you have a better response to insulin. But those who are hypoglycemic doing intermittent fasting now get worse because you're enhancing your hypoglycemia. You have to unwind hypoglycemia first. Once you manage your blood sugar and urinalysis proves you are in ketosis, now you can expect the benefits if IF. You want to skip your breakfast because it gives you more time to fast, but every other day. The result is your blood sugar spikes being stabilized because insulin responds faster and is more efficient. What intermittent fasting (IF) does is it kicks in your metabolism. Sometimes IF gets combined with low calorie intermittent fasting. That's all relative to where you are in your health. If you have any factors that would make this not safe, don't do IF. In our office, we use several programs to get someone into ketogenesis. Either rapidly by a fast mimicking one-week program Prolon program, or a long-term anti-inflammatory ketogenic program. Sometimes you need one or the other or both. I prefer using these before going full blown into ketogenic or IF. But IF can be combined with the anti-inflammatory ketogenic program to maximize your chemistry. [281] [282] [283]

CHAPTER 10

The Toxins Around Us and Between Your Ears

We are exposed to a lot of toxins in our world. Toxins come in many different forms. Most of us are aware of pesticides, heavy metals, herbicides, fungicides, and industrial cleaning solvents. But, toxins come in foods, especially GMO. They come in the air we breathe, the carpets, paint, and cleaners of our homes. Or, when we drive our cars, enter a building that is being refinished or an old building with asbestos. There are also plants that are toxic to touch and what we breathe from them. There are even toxic relationships and thoughts. The bottom line is, we need not live in fear of being exposed to toxins. You are on a daily basis. But, you need to limit what you can so that your body can express its potential.

Not having a good removal system of waste can affect how you sleep or create insomnia every now and then. That is the true measure of your fluctuation. If we can't detoxify, we have imbalance in hormones, fatigue, and weight gain. Toxins also increase temperature. That said, the people who tend to have the most insomnia are often functional at a higher temperature. Your body drops its temperature at night when you sleep. This helps to release sleep-related neurotransmitters. These turn on sleep related hormones so that you can sleep. Should you have trouble sleeping, you might consider a cool pillow or cooling sheets, or even lower the temperature in your home before you go to bed. It's an easy start.

For toxic chemicals in the body, you get glutathione depletion. Losing this can results in a loss of self-tolerance. Then, a reduction in T-regulatory cells to regulate the immune system. This leads to an increase in autoreactive cells and attack your own DNA. You can have chemicals bind to proteins and become chemical sensitivity. Toxins then increase oxidative stress and they decrease mitochondria function thus decreasing energy. They add to intestinal, lung, and brain permeability. In other words, leakiness. This sets up inflammation, disease and autoimmunity reactions. You need to do some necessary steps to reduce them. Using an infrared sauna with all three wavelengths is a great start because you can't avoid everything.[284] [285] [286]

There are a few definitions that will help you understand toxins better. Dose-dependent toxicity is what a lot of manufactures use to label a chemical or drug "safe." This means that for the dose or exposure recommended, there appear to be no adverse health risks.

Dose-dependent, as in the case of caustic chemicals, are labeled harsh as one dose can cause inevitable harm without protection.

The other option that most people are unaware of is a build-up model of toxicity. Over time, a low dose quantity is considered very safe. After continued exposure, the chemical is increasing its concentration into your body. This can build up to a significant quantity that is now harmful to your body and is a toxic dose. This dose can lead to reactions and illness even though you were careful and using the "safe" recommended dose. These doses can affect hormone levels, thyroid function, and autoimmune conditions. [287] [288] [289] [290] [291]

Electromagnetic Field

I will start with the toxins we can't seem to get away from, EMF. Scientists have already observed that EMF (electric and magnetic field) radiation from 5G can penetrate human skin up to 1/64 of an inch. And that 5G radiation penetrates skin more than any other type of radiation currently emitted from our consumer electronics. While 1/64 of an inch may not sound like much, the physical consequences could be dire. The body's response to high frequency radiation involves the parasympathetic system. This can influence pulse rate, perspiration, and blood pressure. This is how you pee, poop, procreate, have immunity, regulate blood sugar and blood supply. It's rather important and is now being disrupted.

In addition, EMF radiation may cause effects at the cellular level, thereby impacting chromosomes, DNA, proteins, and genes. And, the concentration of radio frequency radiation from sub-terahertz waves in skin could yield an unusual result: a sensation of heat and a "sudden, acute pain response. In other words, the sensation would be that of a painful burn even though the skin has not been heated. Look into radiation poisoning and you will find similar changes in the skin. That's scary. [292] [293] [294]

There are quite a few differences between 4 and 5G. The biggest one is the frequency bands. 4G is between 700-2100 micro hertz while 5G is between 28-50 gigahertz. That's the difference in sitting in front of a 1990s calculator watch compared to 4 microwaves bombarding you with radiation! It's more than just going from 4G to5G.

What the early studies are showing as it doesn't make you sick today, it creates an inflammatory response in your brain. When that occurs, it allows the blood brain barrier to open, which is something we don't want. For those who are underdeveloped, and especially young children, they don't have the same amount of density in their skulls. Those who have osteopenia or osteoporosis have less dense skulls. Thicker or denser skulls would slow down EMF when holding the phone to their head. These individuals have more issues with EMS, and that's why I am an advocate for EMF blockers in your house and on your devices.[295] [296]

Chemicals

We live in a more toxic world more than ever before. There were hundreds of chemicals that didn't exist 40 years ago. Not only is research finding these in food and our water, it's even going across the umbilical cord blood before a child is born! Currently there are 84,000 cleared toxins the market deemed safe. [297]It is estimated a few hundred of those have even been tested for safety. Toxicity is a waste that builds up over time in your body. It's comparable to too much exercise, or eating the wrong things for a long period of time, or drinking too much. You know what that feels like. It is important to enhance your detoxification to be able to get rid of waste because it minimizes exposure to your environment. When detoxification pathways are inhibited, this leads to inflammation. And now, you have trouble with your genes methylating. You have trouble making energy, blood supply, and worse. You have trouble with brain function and immunity. Methylation can help this but you need more than food and supplements.

Part of detoxifying your homes to make sure you have a very good air quality and you want to make sure that the humidity in your home remains below 55%. It appears to be the magic number to keep mold in check. I advise you to go by the community measuring device. They're very inexpensive. Put it in the very center of your house. If you're looking for an air purifier, there's a testing organization called Intertek. They set the standard called clean air delivery rate, and you will want over 300. For some guidance for air, cleaning solutions, detergent, and soaps, see the references at the end of this book.

Foods for Detoxification

There are natural foods to help heal your gut such as artichoke, onions, asparagus, and avocados. They have high amounts of sulfur. You can also purchase teas that are specific for detoxification. Or take supplements such as glutathione, NAC, and whey protein isolate to help your body detoxify.

Plastics

You need to be aware of plastic bottled water because a lot of water has what's called BPA. Most bottled water contains phthalates.

Many canned foods and beverages also contain bisphenol A. BPA is an endocrine disruptor and affects hormone function. It's bad enough where the EPA required all child toys and pacifiers to be BPA free. Unfortunately, that is about as far as the ban goes. It still has adverse effects on toddlers, adolescents, and adults. [298] [299]

They will label the outside if they do not. If no label, assume it does. Also, eating foods that are packaged in plastic, or heating them up in plastics is a great way to add a toxic load. Many people microwave on a paper plate. If you've ever thrown a paper plate on an open fire, it doesn't burn like other paper. Black smoke billows out of it. Because it's part plastic. Microwave plastics and you eat plastics. It's not toxins alone. Plastics are hormone disruptors.[300] [301] The real name is xenohormones. To your body a plastic straw with cola being sucked through it is the same as an estrogen pill. For men, that means man boobs. For women they irregular periods, hot flashes, cramps, and migraines to name a few. How many people get a hot coffee in the morning with a plastic lid? That lid drips plastic into your warm latte. Take it off. Or better yet, take a ceramic cup and pour it into something safe.

Water

If you have to buy water on the road, try to purchase from glass bottles. At home, if you have a reverse osmosis system, it can help reduce toxins. Even better is a multistage reverse osmosis system. There are better filtration systems available. It all depends on how much you want to spend. You can always start with some basics and build as you go. You can have everything for a cost. I recommend you prioritize what is important. If you exercise a lot, don't have a filtration system, or live in an apartment or rent a home, you can't put in a filtration system. So, buy a filter for the tap, or a filtration container, and start there.

Living Space

The same goes in your home. If you can put in hardwood floors, do it. When you rent, find tile or hardwood versus carpet because there are so many toxins in carpet. If you have a home, find a space to store your toxic cleaning materials, solvents, and home maintenance. Leaving them in an area that gets hot can vaporize the materials and they can aerosol and you can inhale them. So let's say you have them in a hot garage. And now every time you go to your vehicle, you're exposed. If when you open a cabinet or drawer and a strong scent of the product is present, you're being exposed. While this isn't so bad if your detoxification system works, it can be a disaster if you have health problems, autoimmunity, or recent brain trauma.

Brain Pain

For concussions and other brain trauma, there is a test where we can evaluate the blood brain barrier to see how it's doing. For the immediate future, there is a saliva test that picks up if you are making antibodies to the barrier proteins. Specific to the brain, we use products that help what's called the glyco lymphatic portions of the brain. These contain food for the microglial. If you recall, the microglial system has nine times as many cells than neurons or brain cells. The glyco lymphatic cells clean the brain up and remove metabolic waste. That's detoxification for your brain.[302] [303] [304]

Food Allergy Testing

And if they do have a positive brain barrier test, sometimes the foods that we eat for gut repair are beneficial to help repair the blood brain barrier. Why? The brain, gut, lungs, and sinuses are all barrier systems. When you build one, you build the others. If you have a lot of food sensitivities and chemical sensitivities, you may be in a toxic situation. They may not be the most important of all your sensitivities, but they add up. Understanding what you can eliminate to reduce your toxic load can help your liver, kidney, skin ,and other detoxification organs play catch up.

And then I get the question about coffee: should we drink it, should not drink it? Well, there are certain genes that allow people to eliminate caffeine and break it down. These people can consume caffeine. Dark coffee has some of the best antioxidants out there. There are genes that don't allow people to break down caffeine. Those people have to avoid it. But like things that are beneficial, you can overdo it. So, if you're drinking coffee all day long or you put a lot of sugar in it, you're unlikely to gain any benefit. If you're not sleeping well and you're drinking coffee late in the evening, well, that is an easy fix. In the morning, coffee is a stimulant and it helps make the gallbladder contract, which helps with motility and digestion. For many, it helps them have a bowel movement. This is detoxification 101. If you're not defecating 2-3 times a day, then you are toxic to your own fecal material.

Toxic Stress and Thought Patterns

Does thought affect health, and can you think yourself sick or healthy? Of course. That is called the placebo effect. Not always does a placebo work or is tested in clinical trials. If you break your leg and don't have it set right, I'm not sure how you can think it back into place. There could be a chance you can, and it's my mindset that needs altered. I tend to lean towards reasonable expectations when setting goals that can be achieved. Many American's want a full recovery in two weeks for less than $20. When 75% of us have autoimmune antibodies, that's unreasonable. What is reasonable is a plan for when your brain fog improves or when you have less pain, or your diarrhea, or constipation are now managed. You're able to go back to work, or be the mother you wanted. There should be timelines to get you there and what to change if they do not.[305]

For your body, you need to find a way to reduce stress. Evaluate junk in versus junk out. Junk thoughts or listening to bad music is reflected in how you function, both emotional and chemical functions. Now, bad music, that could be personal. What I'm responding to are brain studies. Take a child in their early development. Do you have them listen to classical music? Or hardcore rap and heavy metal? We all know the answer. There is a wealth of information on how classical music has different tones and helps support different parts of the brain. Yes, a solid repeated rap beat can develop a part of the brain. But if the lyrics are causing negative emotions like hate and anger, how is that helpful for stress? That can be toxic.[306]

These tests go further to show how you digest, think, grow, and fall apart based on the type of music you choose to listen to. Remember, the body only knows stress, it will not identify if it's good or bad. So, if your music, exercise, diet, work, relationship, and home life are stressful, your body responds in reaction to stress. Your body keeps count of each stressful event like a savings account. If you make more withdrawals than deposits, when you make more withdrawals, which one will spiral you towards disease? That is the question to which I have a magic 8 ball in my office. Shake it a few times and it will give you the best answer because it's hearsay. The answer is, who can know?

What we do know is chronic stress is a big cause of irritable bowel, anxiety, and hyperactivity in children. It can also slow down growth and how your immune system works. Stress doesn't have to be finances, work load, sleep, or environment. It can be physiological, like chronic inflammation, or a bad relationship with a partner or parent. [307] [308] [309]

On one hand, I have an uncle who smokes three packs of cigarettes a day and rarely eats. He sticks to black coffee and looks very healthy. Is he? And then there's someone who works out, eats organic, and does all the right things, yet they can't digest anything and look sick.

There is a difference with these two individuals in epigenetic expression with specifics to methylation and detoxification. At some point, and I don't know when, my uncle's habits will catch up to him. And the other, we must continue to adapt and try new things until something works. In case I haven't detailed what can cause stress, there are several types:

•A decrease in joint movement is counterproductive for the immune system (lack of movement stress)

•Heat is good for irreversible arthritis but not most joints with inflammation (Inflammatory stress)

•Physical: "I've fallen and I can't get up." (Overtraining, trauma stress.)

•Mental (Career, kids, mental stress.)

•Emotional (Family, relationships, emotional stress)

•Chemical (Medications, diet, toxins, chemical stress)

There are mental and emotional techniques that are beneficial to your mental state, and these are classes or courses you can take. Ho'oponopono teaches "I'm sorry, please forgive me, I love you." Emotional freedom technique is a stress reduction where you tap acupuncture points while stating affirmations. QI Gong works on the neuro emotional movement of Qi. Neuro Emotional Technique asks questions to your conscious and subconscious through muscle testing. More medical is Eye Movement Desensitization and Reprocessing (EMDR) and also neurofeedback. There is a caveat. If you have too much stress or aren't stable with blood sugar, inflammation, and other physiological states, EMDR can get you down and out for a few days. It works, but you must know about these side effects before starting.

Many of these teach emotions are lies, they are not rooted in truth or grounded in fact. Emotions are distractions from our purposes and can lead to negative thoughts. Let me take an extreme example of fear following the September 11 attacks.

Some ground soldiers were under attack. They were paralyzed from moving for fear of being shot. This is a normal human response. The problem was if they didn't move, they would be flanked and their fear revealed. And if they moved, they might have their fear proven true. But, in the exact moment what they are fearing is not happening to them. Our troops are taught to take a deep breath, slow things down, and think what the best option is. You need to do the same thing in your world. You have worry, fear, and hesitation. None of these are literal and causing you immediate physical harm and pain. But they could. Or doing nothing could also as well..Breath, think, plan, believe, and do.

Understand the most powerful drug is your belief. Then Expect to get better. Expect to come through. Expect this of you. That is why the placebo effect is part of science. It creates real outcomes ,positive or negative.

I will conclude this section with some negative thoughts or language that are detrimental to health. Whether you say this of yourself, of another person, or someone says it to you, I can promise it isn't helpful. If it's you, reword it and make a positive spin. If someone says it to you, do the same. Reword it and make it a positive spin.

Negativity: "Not this person again." Spin: "Nice to see you."

Judgement: "That pain she has is her own fault" Spin: "That's unfortunate. I hope she finds the source of her clumsiness."

Fear: "What if I don't get better?" Spin: "I will get better."

Doubt: "This won't help." Spin: "This will help."

Worry: "If I don't get $300 by tomorrow, I can't pay for my mortgage." Spin: "I can figure out money problems. It's easier than solving world peace."

Negative language: "Well, let's try and see. This is going to take some time. You won't ever recover. I can't help you." Spin: "Let's do this with the expectation of this response."

Here is some positive language from a doctor (but you can apply this for other scenarios):

"It's a good thing you came to see me."

"Come on in, let's get you out of pain, better, or find what you're seeking."

"You are going to feel a difference by tomorrow morning."

"Your body has incredible power to heal."

"Of course, I treat ABC conditions, and you will get great results."

There are doctors who have negative language. If they don't expect you to get better, why are you seeking their advice?

In summary, there are a few things to consider with detoxification from chemicals, environment, and relationships. If you choose products with the least amount of ingredients, you are more apt to make a better choice. Added fragrances and colorings in household products are toxic to many people as are flavor or fragrance on labels. Many manufactures use the words "natural" or "organic" but nature is very good at making poisons. Mold and the coca leaf are poisonous and toxic but are natural and organic. Labels that have "other ingredients" or "spices" are finding a way around the system to get consumers to buy. If you find "non-toxic, petroleum-free, paraben-free," then you have a much safer item.

With paints and solvents, because you have to paint or repair wood in your home at some time, non-VOC or low-VOC is recommended. These are lower risk for depleting your ultra-important glutathione. This is the same for air fresheners. An alternative is essential oils. There are diffusers for these. Yet, this may not be enough. If you have lost your immune-tolerance, they can still make you feel awful. Also, essential oils are an aerosolized fat that coats and goes into everything around them. I recommend keeping them contained in a small area. Not all essential oils are created equal. Some have toxic elements that counteract their effect. Or they like many herbal formulas, the soil and how they are grown make a difference on their function.

Added improved air quality at home includes a system with HEPA filters. Your vacuum needs to have one too. If you are not too close to smog or traffic, open the windows from time to time. Inside plants such a Peace Lily, English Ivy, Chrysanthemum, and Sansevieria help absorb toxins in the air. Keep your humidity below 55% to keep mold from growing and/or add a dehumidifier if you have the option to control it yourself.

CHAPTER 11

Introduction to Acupuncture: A Basic Introduction to Muscle Testing, Meridian Therapy, and Electronics

A cupuncture is defined as a health science used to successfully treat the both pain and dysfunction of the body. One can use standard muscle testing as a basis for testing acupuncture points. It is a principal, not a technique. Many methods can be used to stimulate an acupoint with its main goal to achieve balance.

Acupuncture methods are used to treat over 2,000 conditions and diseases. There are 71 known meridians that energy transverses in your body. Twelve meridians are considered main meridians for which in our office we test and check daily. These energy systems named after the organ system provide function and that can be mapped, tested, and corrected. We use a device known as an Acugraph that works by evaluating the energy traverses of the 12 meridian channels. There are several ways to test the acupuncture system including, but not limited to, pulse points, reflexology, electro meridian imaging, or meridian muscle testing. Electro Meridian imaging is a diagnostic tool that replaces the subjective doctors' findings with an FDA approved electro meridian imaging test. Electro Meridian imaging, otherwise known as meridian graphing and seen below, shows deficiencies and excesses within meridians and well as five-element options to provide a consistent test basis to evaluate the energy of each individual. The goal of acupuncture is a balance between these meridians. Using a combination of 361 main acupoints on the 12 meridians, you stimulate to get balance in your body. If there is a disruption in this energy flow, this can alter the system, producing pain, or symptoms in the body. Meridians are not palpable or observable to the naked eye, but they exist. Through radio isotyping, it was proven these points exist. I hope those test subjects are doing well. They had to submit to radiation to show that these points did exist!

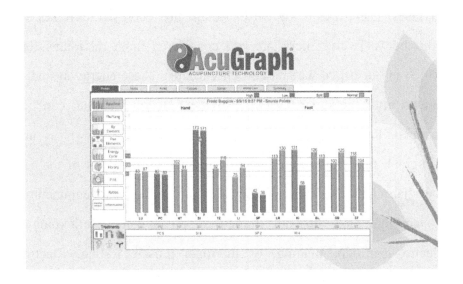

Pulse points consist of evaluating the radial artery in both hands over three finger widths beginning at the wrist. Each pulse point has a deep (yin) or superficial (yang), point for a total of 12 spots corresponding to the 12 meridians. Depending on the pulse itself, strong or weak, and a myriad of other options, this will tell the practitioner if there is excess or deficient energy in the meridian and what to evaluate. These can take 20 years to learn and be efficient in using.

Reflexology points are holographs of the body located in many remote parts that can be treated to ease a condition elsewhere. There are many holographic indexes in the body, but the hands, feet, ears, tongue, and cranium are the most widely used. When a part of the body becomes distressed, there are other connections via the fascia and nervous system that cause irritation in remote parts of the body. These can be treated in a different place, a reflex, to help a particular condition.

Acupuncture research helps the nervous system. It is one the best therapies to balance parasympathetic and sympathetic. It helps cardiovascular conditions and has a positive effect on heart rate variability. Acupuncture has some of the best outcomes with helping people through an opioid addiction. Why are we not using this more? [310] [311] [312] [313] [314] [315] [316] [317] [318]

Indicator muscle tests correlate with individual meridian therapy. Each muscle in the body has an associated meridian connector. For example, if one has chronic tight hamstrings, low back pain, and/or knee pain, this could be a correlation that there is a large intestine problem. Because of the speed, ease, and cost, muscle testing is good for individuals who wish not to afford expensive equipment. But what if your muscles are inflamed? What if you have Fibromyalgia? Those muscles and the testing of them could be skewed. It is because of false negative and positive variables we use a device known as an Acugraph to graph the meridians. Also, their software compares each treatment to evaluate progress. For the doctor using an Acugraph, wouldn't you think it best to know what to treat, how to treat, and if they are getting better? It is my belief that anyone using acupuncture needs to use an Acugraph in their office. I don't understand why anyone who performs this type of acupuncture does not use one.

The history of acupuncture in the United States began when in 1972 President Nixon traveled to China. During his trip, he underwent an emergency appendectomy whereas the anesthesia used were needles instead of medications.

In 1973, the International Acupuncture Meridian Association was created in the United States. It took a while to accept, but in 1995, the FDA classified acupuncture needles as medical instruments and assured their safety and effectiveness. Furthermore, in 1997, the National Institutes of Health (NIH) acknowledged acupuncture as a useful and less adverse treatment to many conditions including, but not limited to, acute and chronic conditions. When there are acute problems, and there has been little or no organ system or tissue damage, the results from acupuncture are often rapid and permanent. For chronic conditions, symptoms may recur from time to time depending on the severity of the chronicity. [319]

When one incorporates kinesiology, results are accentuated for both conditions. Why? Because there are multifactorial ways to treat, evaluate, and correct such problems. Remember, from above, not all kinesiology is perfect, but you can look at many reflexes, muscles, thoughts and other symptoms to test a meridian. This is important if you don't have $2,500 to buy an Acugraph.

There are many ways to stimulate an acupuncture point. Acupuncture itself is a misnomer as it states puncture in the skin. Yet, energy can puncture the skin from light, pressure, and other non-penetrating devices. There are as many as 33 ways to stimulate an acupuncture point. Needles are what most people think. But tapping, lasers, mirrors, magnets, tei shins, and holding via acupressure, are wonderful ways to stimulate points without needles. In fact, it's called needless acupuncture and you can do this at home.

Below are some options to help you save time with evaluating someone. When one stimulates Tsing points, these located on the fingers and toes, they can help musculoskeletal and tendon problems, or even when you don't know what to do. These are tender to press into and the name correlates with someone singing out in pain when a needle is used. Also, stimulation of the four great points of acupuncture- LI 4, Lu 7, Bl 57, St 36 can do a great deal to restore balance. If you are pregnant, omit ST36.

Tsing Points
(Jing-Well Points)

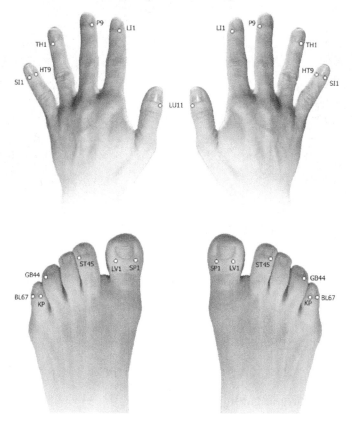

In the event you walk into a room and can't remember why you're there or you need to remember something for yourself, in the morning, K27 will help to connect the left and right brain hemispheres and enable you to think.

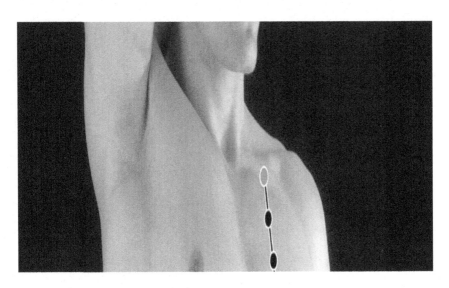

K27 Acupuncture Point

The best option, of course, is memorization of all acupuncture points, muscle testing procedures, or use of advanced testing methods, then interpreting the data provided. I will provide shortcuts and easier options so you don't have to spend years in school and a fortune gaining knowledge.

Advanced Kinesiology Methods

There are a few helpful aides when monitoring muscles via kinesiology methods. Muscle weaknesses create predictable postural alterations, and the problem is that you will usually find multiple weaknesses. Consequently, you will rarely see the indications of a single muscle weakness pattern.

It is a great idea to observe yourself or your family member during motions such as walking, rising from a sitting position, raising the arm, or testing in a position that has caused concern such as sitting ,or in a painful position. There are 639 muscles, 206 bones, and millions of ligaments, tendons and other connective tissue pathways in the human body. Muscles and ligaments provide the foundation for the transfer of tensile forces throughout the structure. These structures maintain integrity by a continuous balance of tensile forces similar to a stack of bricks. Muscles act as cables to stabilize the joint. This is why they get so tight with injury or inflammation. These tensile forces create balance in the skeletal structure, and the force is then transferred from the muscle and ligamentous structures, then to the periosteum (skin of the bone) for balance and support.

Many individuals have had knee, hips, disc, and shoulder replacement. What about muscles? Medicine has a history of replacing the joint or structure, compromised by an imbalanced force through the joint or structure. Basic structural balance is achieved along lines of tensile force throughout the body. Lines of force create myofascial meridians, who allow the transfer of force from soft tissue, muscles, and ligaments, to the osseous structure, bones, back to the soft tissues. If I'm speaking way too medical, let me help you along.

Look up "Bodies in Motion." These people donated their bodies to science. Most of the skin and bones are gone in these models. The remaining fascia, made of muscles and connective tissue, still holds the model in place. This is called myofascial.

Reactive muscles work in a chain. If you have a reactive muscle in your foot, then you could have one in your shoulder because there is a fascial chain connecting both. Tensile forces of the myofascial planes help to create balance to achieve proper function at both the cellular and energetic levels. Myofascial planes transfer their force to the fascia of the organs and further down the extracellular matrix (ECM) to the base structure of the tissue. ECM forces are transferred into the membrane matrix of the cell membrane. The cellular function is dependent upon the larger tensile forces that are transferred from the myofascial planes to the ECM integrins. These are otherwise known as connections between the ECM and a cellular wall. An imbalance is actually transferred into the nucleus of a cell where the DNA is held and can change cell function, allowing for a disturbance in energetic function. This is the fundamentals of genetics. It defines epigenetic expression. You can put imbalances or changes as environmental, food, lifestyle, and exercise. These changes can lead to potential precursors for pathology or disease. It's both biochemical and energetic.

Introduction to Muscle Testing Kinesiology

What is Kinesiology? It's a neurological test for biomechanics, balance, function, range of motion, a measurement of body, mind, and chemical health. Although many speak of body "energy," we are more so dealing with the nervous system. More importantly, brain function. All the changes observed are monitored and mediated through the nervous system. When someone trained is performing clinical kinesiology, they are looking for functional short circuits which can be corrected as opposed to "dead" circuits of the body. Dead circuits are out of a natural or conservative scope of practice. An example may be diabetic neuropathy where the nervous system is no longer communicating with the body. Another example: There are muscles associated with organ-related energy systems to be explained below. These imbalances could state pathology, a neurological condition, an emotional condition, a lack or excess of a nutrient, or an injury.

Below is a list of muscles and associated organ or organ energy systems

•Lung > Serratus anterior

•Large Intestine > Tensor fascia latae

•Stomach > Pectoralis major, clavicular division

•Spleen/Pancreas > Latissimus Dorsi

•Heart > Subscapularis

•Small Intestine > Quadriceps

•Bladder > Peroni group

•Kidney > Psoas

•Circulation Sex > Gluteus medius

•Triple Warmer > Teres minor

•Gall Bladder > Popliteal

•Liver > Pectoralis major, sternal division

As you can see, there is a connection between the muscle and the organ. This is not only through the nervous system, but also through the energy of a functional human being. There are many different elements being monitored by muscle testing that it can only be hypothesized on its effects. There are many people who muscle test and consider it kinesiology, but is it? How many people do it well? In my humble opinion, based on knowledge of functional testing, not as many as one would hope, more like less than ten percent.

We can all make thoughts in our heads and perceive a weakness or strength, swaying or stability, be content or in distress. Let me elaborate on creating a physiological response based on thought alone. Do you remember my lemon analogy in the middle of a desert where you're very parched? Most of you created physiology called saliva through thought. Turn on the TV and you'll see plenty of thought-provoking ads. When you create physiology from thought, you have performed quantum physics on yourself. You have taken yourself out of the realm of conventional science and into alternative medicine. From this process you need to decide what is correct for you.

A standard muscle testing is the basis for kinesiology and one common factor is observed: weak to strong and strong to weak. Learning how to test subtle changes in muscles will be a lifelong learning experience as each individual is different in health, biochemistry, strength, and function. Many muscle testing technicians use the arm pull-down test. Is this adequate, precise, and infallible? No. Nothing is perfect and the precision of an arm pull-down test is far from precise as over 20 muscles could be brought into the test. At best, it's adequate in a time of haste.

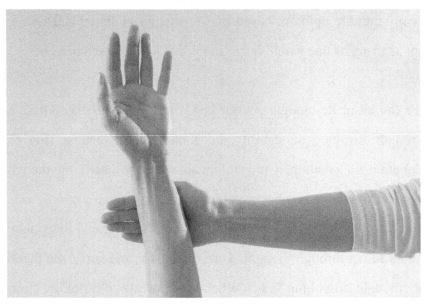

What does a change in muscle strength mean? It could mean nothing, fatigue, toxic, deficient, change in metabolic demand, etc. So, the practitioner needs to have some working knowledge of the anatomy, physiology, and of course the nervous system. If it's an organ, muscle, or nerve pathway, which fibers does it follow and where does it land in the brain? If there is a weakness without, what does that mean? Are there blood tests to substantiate an organic or nutritional weakness? Is there a stressor or mechanoreceptor out of balance?

I absolutely love kinesiology but you can see why there are so many different answers for a weak or strong muscle. We really need to know the frequency that is impacting the muscle fiber, it's source, and where and how to fix the pathway. That is when you are performing or receiving kinesiology-based methods at its best. Of course, medical testing to backup findings keeps the practitioner honest and the patient compliant.

There are some rules with muscle testing. One must test the individual muscles indicated through the 12 meridians on both sides of the body. Although many speak of body "energy," we are ultimately dealing with the nervous system, most importantly, brain function. All the changes observed are monitored and mediated through the nervous system. We are looking for functional short circuits that can be readily corrected as opposed to "dead" circuits of extreme pathology.

Kinesiology allows us to evaluate too little or too much energy. It's neuroanatomy at its best where the communication between the brain and its circuitry yields an explosion in knowledge. One common factor is a change in muscle strength, inhibition versus facilitation. Is it communicating or not? Too much or not enough nerve energy leads to disease. No matter what you change, the final common pathway to a muscle is the anterior horn motor neurons to that muscle. It's neurological or mechanistic, but it's also chemical, physiological, and energetic. That's how you can test function neuroanatomy and basic physiology. We are looking for short circuits, which can be corrected. Muscle testing equals functional neurological evaluation. Alternative muscle evaluation equals alternative muscle testing which is functional neurological evaluation.

There are two main types of muscle tests. First, Gamma I, where the tester begins the test. This is a spinal reflex and does not go to higher centers in the brain with testing. The tester will push first or hit with a reflex hammer and see how the individual responds. Secondly, with Gamma II, the individual begins the test. This test goes to higher centers in the brain and gives better neurological information to the tester because one has to think to contract.

Rules for muscle testing that can help with precision and when you should walk away from a treatment. The practitioner must:

• Approximate the origin and insertion of the muscle

- Stabilization of the joint the muscle crosses

- Contact with the soft parts of your testing hand

- Instruct the person being tested to push in the required direction

- Increase the force slightly

- Repeat any test when one is not quite sure with a muscle test

- Use different muscles when the strong indicator become fatigued

- Not muscle testing EVERY person in your family at least once because necessity is the mother of all invention.

How mistakes are made with muscle testing:

- Not informing the person a test is going to be performed

- Bouncing

- Joints and joint placement. For example, a bent elbow

- Crossing a joint while testing

- Not placing the subject in a testable position

- Not testing in the correct posture

- Allowing for the subject to touch an injured tissue inadvertently

- Testing on different sides of the body, not being consistent with testing protocol

- Not being consistent with other joints

Microcurrent

There is also a need to understand infrasonic versus auditory frequencies. Infrasound frequencies are lower than the human hearing threshold of 20 hertz. Humans can perceive frequencies below this but not particularly be aware by hearing or feeling. Some of these infrasonic frequencies are found in thunderstorms, geomagnetic storms, earthquakes, jet streams, mountain ranges, rocket launchings, and weather patterns. These infrasonic frequencies can travel long distances and be measured hundreds of miles away. Research shows that mammals understand and perceive those signals and humans do too. Technology, such as microcurrent and some forms of biofeedback, neuro modulation, and other sub auditory frequencies are infrasonic. These technology options can affect physiology such as heart rate variability, hearing, inflammation, and many other actions on nerve fibers. They can also come in harmonics both inaudible and auditory.

Auditory frequencies are variable on the health, age, and inflammatory conditions of an individual, and what is perceived through the ear. More exact, how the cilia or hair of the ear vibrate with the inner ear bones. This vibration with the hair tells the brain what is being perceived. Damage to that area of the brain, or the inner ear bones, or the hair, can have a marked decrease in hearing and the ability to hear auditory frequencies.

Microcurrent is the application of frequency-specific electrical currents to the injured part of the body. Microcurrent therapy helps injured tissue heal faster and provides relief from pain caused by injury or chronic conditions. Microcurrent uses low-voltage electricity to stimulate muscle, adenosine triphosphate (ATP) cell growth, and collagen development in the dermis on the face. There are quite a few devices for a non-surgical facelift based on micro current technology. This isn't new technology. Microcurrent has been around for decades, especially in physical therapy, so it is very safe, effective, and targeted because you can use frequency-specific therapy for individual tissues and conditions. These conditions include pain, inflammation, swelling, infections, brain function, bone, wound healing, muscle function, allergies, and much more. 320 321 322 323 324 325 326 327 328 329 330 331 332 333 334 335 336 337 338 339 340 341 342 343 344 345 346 347 348 349 350 351 352 353 354 355 356 357 358 359

The confusion is microcurrent is like TENS devices. TENS deliver milliamp current and block pain messages that are trying to get up the spine to the brain. Micro-current delivers sub-sensory micro amperage current, 1000 times less than milli-amperage current, which has been shown in published studies to increase ATP production in tissues. It's relatively safe, but if you are pregnant, have epilepsy, a pacemaker, metallic inserts on the treatment sites, or are an insulin dependent diabetic, you are not a candidate. Regardless, my biased opinion from the fantastic results I've observed over the years is why I am working on a home device so everyone has access to the benefits of microcurrent. It won't fix everything, but it can make you feel better. Perhaps that's enough to work a few more hours. Or, it's enough pain relief to reduce medications with dangerous side effects. These and many other reasons either save money or allow you to create money with a home device.

What is frequency-specific microcurrent? Frequency-specific microcurrent (FSM) is a technique for treating pain by using low-level electrical current. In using FSM to treat pain, it's been found that various frequencies can be used to potentially reduce inflammation (swelling), repair tissue, and reduce pain. Is it different for microcurrent? Yes and no. It's still a microcurrent but the user can change the frequencies at will, so it has more uses. Some devices only come with 3-5 pre-programmed frequencies. Are those frequency-specific? Yes. They are just limited on how many are available to the user. [360] [361] [362] [363]

Currently there is a minimum of research that began in the late 70's regarding microcurrent. PubMed has hundreds of research with improvement in pain of 80-90%. That's awesome. The original micro-current was a derivative of a transdermal electro neuro stimulation (TENS) device with a specific programming versus estimated phases, bandwidth, and frequency. Initial devices could pre-program polarity and frequency for thought conditions, feeding frequency into the body via an electrode or probe. Originally this was thought to be a Rife-like device, but unlike Rife, there are other parameters into play than just frequency. The nervous system is a collection of data and those are collected by specific receptors throughout the body. The brain is responsible for collecting the data, assimilating, and deciding what is important, and what is simply noise. Rife blasts its working knowledge of frequencies all at once to the nervous system with the idea that one of those frequencies is seen as beneficial to the nervous system and thus a positive health improvement response. Advanced microcurrent allows for changes to how the nervous system needs stimulation by adding additional parameters than just frequency. In most muscle stimulation devices, polarity, positive and negative, are a frequent addition. Advanced microcurrents allow for four parameters: frequency, polarity, amplitude, and waveform. It is the addition of the last two parameters that allows microcurrents to pinpoint a direct frequency rather than a shotgun approach to what could be.

Future research will be combining a lab and run pre- and post-inflammatory tests to show its efficacy and get into peer-reviewed periodicals. This will come at some cost, roughly with a point-of-care-testing device (POCT) for one of several of the inflammatory markers, including but not limited to LDL, A1C, Insulin, C-reactive protein, Ferritin, Homocysteine, LDH. Even Cleveland Clinic is promoting microcurrent on their website for treating no less than 20 conditions. Now you know, microcurrent is here.

There are already several devices in several sectors to reverse engineer. The difficulty will be in finding an engineer that can make it wireless, portable, and user friendly with a professional and home edition, if not an app that can be successful through a smartphone. That way you can observe imbalances in yourself or your family and run energy into your body. Pretty cool, huh?

CHAPTER 12

Mechanoreceptors

I t's all about balance, but in achieving such balance, it is what your mechanoreceptors are telling your brain. What is a mechanoreceptor (MR)? These are specialized sensory receptors that respond to mechanical pressure or distortion. They constantly send signals to your spinal cord and to the brain through what is called afferent (away from) neurons (nerves) through synapses in your cord. The second nerve goes to your thalamus, located in the brain, and the third neuron then goes to the sensory area in your brain called the cortex. These stimuli are communicated on what requires movement or changes in what you are doing to keep you functional.

There are several groups of these MR. Meissner's corpuscles, (light touch and light vibration,) Pacinian corpuscle (rapid vibrations and some internal organs,),and Ruffini ending (skin and fascia tension,) and are linked to muscle activation. Merkel's complex does not, but instead detects sustained pressure. There are also MR in the cochlea of the inner ear and these transduce sound to the brain, and baroreceptors are MR that are excited by the stretching of a blood vessel.

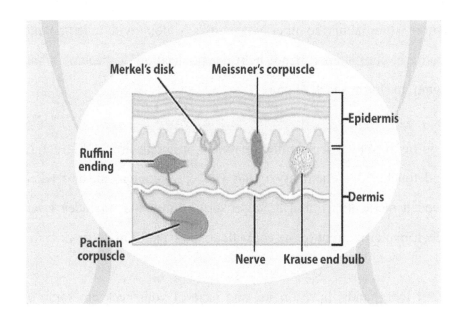

Merkel's disk   Meissner's corpuscle

Epidermis

Ruffini
ending

Dermis

Pacinian
corpuscle

Nerve   Krause end bulb

In our office, we understand that the MR Merkel have small receptive fields that respond to static stimulation and compression of a joint, and Ruffini respond to electricity and muscle stretching. Pancinian respond to low-light laser therapy and electrical vibration, and Meissner's respond to touching of the skin. Just an FYI: If your practitioner is not touching you in any way, can you see how this could slow down your recovery?

There are other receptors for pain (nociception,) temperature, and balance (vestibular). Nociceptors go into the brain and the cord and act as reflexes for pain stimuli so that you move before your brain says "ouch!" Sometimes these can over fire, and the pain does not seem to ever go away. Understanding how the nervous system works, stimulating the other MR pathways along with nutrition and exercise, can dampen if not help the nociceptors to become silent again, meaning a lack of pain.

I do my best to articulate that treatment protocols are 33% structure and touch, 33% chemistry (what you eat, supplement, and when needed medication), and 33% sensory stimuli that includes laser, electric microcurrent or the equivalent and balance brain work.

Your feet, hands, lips, tongue, and base of your neck are some of the biggest concentrations of mechanoreceptors. While your lips and tongue are off-limits in most offices, you have plenty of other surfaces to stimulate at home.

Why would you stimulate? Mechanoreceptor knowledge has more than 50 years of clinical research and outcomes. In my opinion, in speaking to doctors in many fields, many doctors are finding it increasingly more challenging to help patients, and the majority of doctors are not using MR stimulation. This is a big deal. In fact, due to research findings, Harvard Medical University, Yale University, and Cleveland Clinic are incorporating MR stimulation by micro-current—a device we have used in our office starting on my first day of licensure. Why? Because that's what the research shows for better outcomes. 364 365 366 367 368 369 370 371 372

Want to make a big difference on mechanoreceptors? Take a look at your footwear.

Shoes

Let us talk about shoes, yes, I'm talking to you, ladies. I get the importance, the status, the feeling you get with some sweet shoes. I'm not telling you to move to flats or SAS for the remainder of your life. Just make good decisions when and where you use them. If your job requires you to wear heels, and I'm not sure how that's legal. Can you change under your desk, or to and from the office? Do they have to be on the entire time? I used to take new doctors to the mall to watch people. If the heel or shoe is supportive, there is a different response in how people walk—their gait. My favorite way to observe gaits is walking in with ponytails. If the shoe or heel is supportive, the hair will swish from side to side. If not, upon impact, the entirety of the spine is activated like a whip, and the pony tail goes up and down. It's self-induced whiplash!

Shoes are important to your structure, joints, muscles, and ligaments. They can immediately impact your health.

Shoes and arches are important. Other than your brain, the most important body part is your feet. You have numerous ligaments with hundreds and thousands of nervous fiber receptors known as proprioceptors, and very limited musculature. These proprioceptors are responsible for pressure, temperature, and contractile strength. It is common knowledge that we are able to stretch a muscle, and it will not fail unless we overstretch and cause a tear, as muscles resemble rubber bands. Once stretched, they return back to their original mechanistic shape. Ligaments and connective tissue are a different story. They are more like a plastic sack, rigid in its structure with a crystalline matrix surrounding it's outside. This allowed a more efficient transfer of energy, some of this energy is physiological nervous tissue, but the majority is by the piezoelectric effect by the fascia. The fascia holds the acupuncture points. The acupuncture meridians flow into the chakras, and extraordinary meridians are communicated via physiology to allow something as simple as wearing adequate fitting shoes to stop heartburn.

When finding a shoe, there are six steps to choosing your shoes and three steps to create longevity and stability in your shoes. It is important to know that you actually have three arches, but we will focus on the main longitudinal or middle arch. The middle will drop with improper supporting shoes and incorrect lacing. I have a diagram on how to do this proper in the reference section.

How to pick out a functioning shoe:

Length

The first decision is to purchase a shoe of the correct length. The tendency is to have snug-fitting shoes. This will actually increase injuries, illness, fatigue, and depression. Short shoes will turn off 122 muscles! That is roughly 25% of all skeletal muscles can add to increased fatigue, decreased function, and increased illness.

To avoid short shoes, make sure you have at least one thumb width from the end of your shoe to your longest toe (your anatomical thumb). Shoes that taper or bend on the end must be sized from the bend as this actually makes them smaller (think heels). When it comes to shoes, don't assume you have a set shoe size. Always try your shoes on and make sure each side is not touching any malleoli (these are the ankle bones or bumps protruding on both sides of your ankles. A shoe that touches a malleoli will literally tap the bone out of place causing ankle, knee, hip, and opposite shoulder pain.

Counter Durability (Heel)

The counter is responsible for maintaining the many ligaments and supporting your ankle. It must be uniform on both sides and not pushed down or indented from incorrect packaging or storage. Push the back of the shoe in a pinching fashion. If the counter (heel) goes in very far, it will not support the foot. Push the sides of the counter with the same pinching manner. If the sides close together this will once again not support the foot.

Bending at the Widest Point

Take a pen and roll it down to the widest point of your shoe. Make a mark on the side. Push the shoe together at both ends. Did it bend at your mark? Is there a break there? If you answered no, your shoes will hinder your muscle strength, and in time your health.

Uniformity and Design

Look at the back of the shoe. Does the seam come up the back straight? Does it match your Achilles tendon? If not, you have incorrectly fitting shoes. Shoes are not created on the same day in the same city. Measure them heel to heel to assure you are not wearing false orthotics. Air Technology: this isn't just your name brand only, almost all shoe lines have an "Air" line. Air technology is fashionable, but not supportive, especially if you can see it. Without proper support, muscles will contract hard to maintain support and balance. Muscles without rest become fatigued and highly susceptible to injury. A weak air pocket is the same as driving on a flat tire. Something will wear out.

Creating Longevity and Stability in Your Shoes

Avoid buying shoes mail order, if that's going to be possible in our future. You have not tried those shoes on, even if you did at a store. Buy two pairs of the same shoe if you can. One shoe lasts roughly 300 miles before normal breakdown. Rotating two pairs of the same shoe will last about 500 miles. It costs more upfront but you will save more over a year. But, I understand the world has changed. If you must, order two pairs and run the previous tests. In a perfect world, you can at least keep a pair and return the defective ones. So, make sure you have and understand the return policy.

Lace and Unlace Your Shoes

Pulling off shoes or pushing one's toes into the heel and tugging it off creates strain in the ligaments of the foot. You can stretch a muscle and it will heal, but you cannot stretch a ligament. This will also break down your shoe fast! There's an easy way to keep your kids honest by having them purchase their next pair, should they refuse to tie and untie their shoes. Follow the picture in appendix A for the correct lacing pattern. This will help to prevent the dropping of the navicular bone, which sits above the middle longitudinal arch. As you walk, the normal laces will tap this bone. Over time this will allow the navicular to drop causing a fallen arch, which could attribute to knee, hip, and low back pain. FYI: flip flop sandals cause this. Not unlacing your shoes over time will ruin them faster than anticipated.

Here are some other ways to hurt your feet:

-Consistently using heels over 2 inches or "Cinderella" slipper heels, stilettos, or wearing an unstable shoe after strenuous exercise within 48 hours, like running a race.

-Long-term usage of flip flops and using orthotics when unnecessary. If you use orthotics, make sure you have the right ones when you need them. Many people are told they have leg length problems. After thousands of x-rays and research, very few have a true leg length problem, which is anatomical. They are born with it or had a serious accident or injury. Most "leg length" problems are muscular in nature and do not require orthotics or heel lifts, and when they do, it's for a relatively short amount of time.

-Injuries are weak areas prone to repeat. If you get an injury or illness in a particular area, this will be the area of weakness that could be structural, toxins, nutritional deficiencies, emotional, and mental imbalances. Be aware of what you have and give some thought to what happened and what you can do to prevent it from happening again.

How can you perform mechanoreceptor stimulation at home? While there is a separate manual for specific conditions and issues, below is a 30,000-foot approach. At times, it's very effective. When it works, do you need to know why?

You can find any acupuncture point and rub it for about 10-30 seconds. This stimulates the point. Also, vibration, laser, tei shin, and ear seeds are effective to stimulate the point by way of mechanoreceptor stimulation at home for a very low cost.

To be more specific, you can look up an acupuncture point for your condition and rub it, laser it, or put an ear seed on it from the reference manual or online. When you use a laser, there are a few things to know. Acupuncture has been around for thousands of years, but not everyone wants to go out and start sticking themselves to see if they feel better. Laser acupuncture (LA) uses non thermal, low intensity lasers to stimulate acupuncture points. Over the past decade, there are numerous studies on LA as being able to reduce pain, have less treatment time of 10-60 seconds per site versus 15-30 minutes with a needle. It's non-invasive and has the same effects of analgesia.

LA is a form of low-level laser therapy (LLLT,) and in your cell membranes you have an organelle known as the mitochondria. Red light, not blue or green, is absorbed by cytochrome C oxidase protein and associates with increased energy production. This aids in signaling and regulation of nerves and gene expression. Research has also found in vivo effects of low level laser therapy on inducible nitric oxide synthase resulting in better blood supply.[373] [374 375 376 377 378 379 380 381 382]

LLLT protects the cells against several inflammatory pathways that cause cellular death and improve cell physiology though increased cellular respiration. Think of trying to run fast while holding your breath versus being able to take fast deep breaths. That is what cellular respiration is like. LLLT is also important as an antioxidant because it reduces ROS species, a dangerous free radical. These conditions include insulin, pain, skin, stem cells, inflammation,

315

cardiovascular health, erectile dysfunction, and many more conditions. This is all from an easy-to-work laser you can use at home. 383 384 385 386 387 388 389 390 391 392 393 394 395

Lasers come in 4 classes with the first 2 being non-biological and class 4 being hard lasers that cut or coagulate in surgery. Class 3 comes in 2 forms, 3A also known as 3R, and 3B, and the intensity of the beam and its size affect its depth and energy penetration. Both, if shone in the eye, can cause damage and discomfort. Lasers up to 5mW are classified as 3A and 5-500 is 3B. I recommend you get a 3A laser. This is not a typical laser pointer, although you could use it as one, those have completely different wavelengths and do not treat.

Your laser needs to:

-Have the correct 635nM with a 5mW output, the maximum for a 3A laser.
-Contains an on-off switch so you don't have to sit and hold it and the batteries can easily be replaced or can run on rechargeable batteries.
-Is an FDA class IIIa Laser and comes in its own case with all-metal laser encasing that can take an "oops" and continue to function.

-Comes with a fixed focus to keep the same intensity through any moment.

You should be able to click the laser on, shine it on the point, and wait 10-60 seconds. If you're doing a routine stimulation, 10 seconds should be enough. If you have a chronic issue, or something very acute that you are not needing to go to the hospital for, then hold for up to 60 seconds per area. Start at 90 degrees from your skin, and while you can go through clothes, placing it on your skin may have deeper penetration and better results. You may clean with alcohol, but be careful around the diode and make sure to store in the box it came in.

3A laser (pen size) with metal case

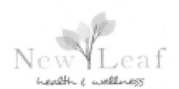

Use of a Tei Shin

While lasers are energy treatments, a tei shin is mechanoreceptor stimulation, you can also use your tei shin to find if you have an active point by pressing it into an acupuncture point. If it's tender, it is most likely active. These are very inexpensive devices to stimulate your body. You can plunge 15 times with the spring end of your device or use the laser. Both work but with different pathways. A tei shin is best for the ear and the hand. The side of the tei shin is effective in rolling on the fingers while the ball on the end can kneed into thicker tissue such as the thumb pad. Also, you can plunge on ear points from auriculotherapy, just be sure not to use it in your ear canal or close to your eye.

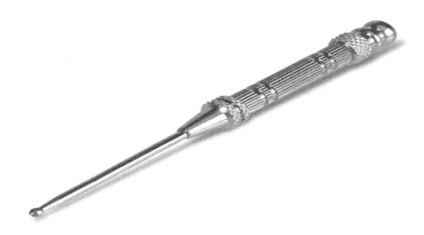

How to Use Ear Seeds

Ear therapy known as auriculotherapy is one of the fastest ways to stimulate the nervous system. Dr. Nogier discovered there are nerve endings that fire into parts of the brain that correlate to the entire body. You can stimulate joints, organs, and nerve bundles all from the ears, and ear seeds are the easiest to use. You can also use the Tei Shin or laser, but ear seeds can remain there for a constant.

There are books, websites, and our self-help manual to better hone in on the points to help yourself. Here's a quick way to find it knowing nothing about the ear or its anatomy.

-Find the point you want to stimulate. If it's tender, it is most likely active but it could be a red or white coloring different from the skin color itself. Ear seeds both activate and suppress, so it doesn't matter which one you need, they do both.

-Peel off the holder. I like to use my tei shin to stick the end and apply on the point. You can use anything that allows you access to your ear.

-A few times a day, reach up and pinch the seed for about 15 seconds. If you have acute pain, you may want to do this hourly or more. Don't push so hard to cause more discomfort than necessary. Seeds are there to suppress pain not irritate. If you have it on a joint, move the affected area, like a shoulder, around while you pinch the seed.

-If they don't fall off the skin in 3 days, take them off as your skin can grow around them. You can always replace them.

Mini-Massager and Other Vibration Tools

These are only intended for reflex points with only one to two pounds of pressure. Using it incorrectly includes using it too long or in the wrong direction. Most importantly, in the wrong location, which is away from the heart. Generally, use a massager on lymphatics tissue and over muscles because they move the lymphatic system.

CHAPTER 13

Putting It All Together

A lthough there are multiple factors allowing conditions of the body to react, two of the more important factors are acidity and lack of oxygen. Too much acidity the systems such as digestion, absorption, immunity, and elimination are inhibited. Lack of oxygen creates a hypoxic condition and the tissue no longer has the ability to heal because it's become acidic. This causes pain by the inflammation pathways provided by hypoxia.

It would be wonderful if physicians began using energetic testing as a method for diagnostics. If a medication caused a potential side effect, the idea is they could catch it before administering it to the patient, or apply it with an electronic, instead of the more dangerous physical entity. This is a thought process with neuro based or micro-current based technology, that one day could be used as a screen process to reduce or understand unwanted side effects. This is why someday in your home you will have a device that uses micro-current either from a hand-held device or a smart phone connected to you.

Science attempts to quantify the nervous system by measuring with EKGs, EEGs, MRIs, and Computer Topography, but is it really what we are? We know that mental thought alone can generate electrical stimulation. Our energy field, being high or low, can shift with those thoughts. Furthermore, there is a high correlation to the cosmos and our interaction with the universe. Ask any police officer or psychiatrist about full moons. Study after study has shown during a full moon there are more admissions to the psychiatric ward and increases in suicides following a waning moon, and an increase in death rates following a full moon. It happens. The EKG, EEG, MRI, and moon are enormous magnets. Your body responds to these.

Magnets are everywhere, including inside you. In the early 1900s, Dr. Thacher formed the Chicago Magnetic Company that used magnets placed on the body or sewn into clothing or shoes to heal. He found that placing the magnets over certain areas of the body could give symptomatic relief for many conditions. There are many companies today relying and selling products that provide similar relief. This does not mean you need to go out and purchase multiple magnets and place them all over your body. The right one in the right location is the best way to make a difference.

In 1954, Linus Pualing received the Nobel Prize in chemistry for his discovery of the magnetic properties of hemoglobin. This is an iron-rich protein molecule that carries blood gasses such as oxygen and carbon dioxide in the blood. Dr. Pauling, through his studies, confirmed some of Thacher's theories that magnets placed in certain places on the body can provide some analgesic relief in some circumstances. Why? The correct magnet could help bring in more blood to a particular area of vascular deficiency.

When hemoglobin passes through a capillary, the magnetic hemoglobin (iron portion) is passing through an electrical neutral collagen-based capillary. This allows its ionic charge holding the hemoglobin to disassociate by way of the opposite charge of the local tissue. On the opposite side of the capillary, the pH of the area allows the re-association of carbon dioxide to the hemoglobin. Then away it goes to the lungs for another energy exchange.

Magnetism begins at the atomic level with small particles known as electrons orbiting around the atom. When all the electrons spin the same way, you get magnetism. Magnetic therapy has been used for centuries from the Greeks to Cleopatra and as far back as 2000 B.C. from Chinese literature.

In the human body, the nervous system communicated via magnetic ions. Cells have paramagnetic fields centered in the DNA. These are produced by the biochemical processing of nutrients, water, and oxygen. There are two poles in every magnet, north or positive, and south or negative. Negative poles calm neurons, encourage relaxation, sleep, ATP formation, and general anesthesia. The opposite positive pole adds stress to the body, produces acidity, and reduces cellular oxygen. The South pole facilitates the spread of microorganisms and stimulation of neurons. Too much of either pole in particular locations results in imbalance. Unfortunately, over time, pathology creates disease processes.

In the late 19th century, Franz Anton Mesmer, a French Physician, used magnetic passes over a patient instead of the placing of magnets. Mesmer noticed there was a correlation between the sun and moon and how that energy of light was thought to be reflected by vibrational light. These observations affected the human nervous system. His theory was that this magnetic force could heal and energize living tissue. Mesmer used permanent magnets for some conditions. But his main treatment consisted of certain hand gestures over the body that were known as "magnetic passes." Often, the passes worked as well as the magnets themselves and he coined "Mesmerized." Over time it was discovered that magnets vibrate at a measurable frequency. Forward to the 21st century.

Now the use of microcurrent combines neurological stimulation with vibration properties.

According to Albert Einstein, time and space are relative, not constant. If you remember Newtonian physics and the physical laws matter abides by? Well, these laws disintegrate in the subatomic realm. Furthermore, there is no difference between energy and matter. We, in turn, live in an infinite sea of energy. Throughout this sea, energy travels in small packets, known as "Quanta." These packets "seem" to be the smallest possible unit of energy or matter. They exhibit intelligence on the micro and macro levels. Quanta defies the laws of Newtonian Physics.

In Newtonian physics, energy can be changed in form, but cannot be created or destroyed. Every action has an equal and opposite reaction. I'm sure you recall hearing that now, but I promise you, this will not be a physics lecture. When an atomic bomb explodes, there is not an equal and opposite reaction. Quanta also defies the laws of thermodynamics. When a Qi Gong practitioner (energy doctor) lays hands on an individual, the master uses the power of thought to treat or heal the patient. At some level, the magnetic vibrations are exact to get the desired effect. Is matter conserved? Is thought matter or is it energy? If the laws of Newtonian physics are applied through the transfer of energy, anyone who lays hands on someone to balance energy in the subject, including all prayer, the transfer of energy would result in a net loss of energy. Thus, resulting in the ill health of those using prayer and the laying of hands to heal.

Because this is not true, those practicing acupuncture, kinesiology (muscle movement and biomechanics), massage, and other therapies are not killing themselves treating people this way.

The use of other alternative medicines, energy healing by definition, cannot bring in or kick out energy. Remember, energy cannot be created or destroyed and needs to have equal and opposite reactions. Energy can be moved and it must to achieve balance and health. Your hands are magnets. You can test each finger for polarity. You were made to heal yourself and be healthy.

Functional Interconnection

If a child is still having trouble with bed wetting, then most likely they are not developing their brain for the part(s) that controls this. There are ways to check for function without expensive radiographic testing, but there are times this is needed. The pathways for autism are the same for ADD, ADHD, depression, anxiety, Parkinson's, and Alzheimer's diseases. So, the tests run for a child should be very similar to an adult with these issues. Also, traumatic brain injuries, a leaky gut, or concussions can all add to these conditions. Autoimmunity, blood sugar being too high (hyperglycemia or diabetes), or too low (hypoglycemia), a faulty gallbladder, or eating bad fats, no fats, or not digesting fats can all lead to the above. As long as you have a heartbeat, you need to understand these pathways and do you best to fight off dementia. I will have webinars about these on our website to explain this better because I would never be able to stop writing with the amount of information available. When you get better with memory or function with autoimmunity or neurodegeneration, understand you are not cured. It's still coming. We have at least slowed down the process. Work, change, make the effort to thwart it as long as possible. Find someone who uses a Right Eye or similar device to evaluate your brain function as well as forms to decipher which part(s) of your brain can benefit from exercises, tasks, skills, and memory games.

When you work on your brain, you will need fuel. It is imperative for you to be able to digest the food you eat. You need to be able to break down your food and you need to have motility. For those that take digestive antacids, proton pump inhibitors and others like it, you have a loss of the first phase of digestion, but most likely you also have a loss of oral tolerance. What this means is that you don't digest the first part of protein, and food particles arrive in your intestines in bulk and not broken down. This can lead to something you will learn about later as permeable membrane, but also immune issues, bloating, heartburn, a sensitive stomach, diarrhea, and constipation. The latter could be more than just a gastrointestinal issue. I bring this up again because of its importance in the nervous system. Chronic constipation can be a sign of Parkinson's disease or other brain dysfunctions. There could also be an autoimmune issue within the nervous system, or more specifically, the enteric nervous system that runs digestion. It could be a lack of fiber or an infection, or a change in your microbiome, the cells that act in synergy to you the host inside your intestines.

Simply supplementing is not the best approach to fix the problem. So many patients come in with bags of supplements and a prayer. They haven't been told they can't digest the majority of what they are taking. Usually, we start with the top, as this top down physiology. We do our best to help with oral tolerance and eliminate any infections, all the while working on brain function to see if we can make a difference.

And now, a final recap. A loss of oral tolerance means a loss of hydrochloric acid. That leads to a loss of insulin tolerance that can lead to diabetes, heart disease, anemia, cancers, autoimmune diseases, and brain issues such as Alzheimer's and Parkinson's diseases. It's a big deal.

Electromagnetic energy is part of the human body. It can produce illness and help to bring in healing depending on its strength. The ground we walk on each day is magnetic. The Earth is magnetic through its magma, and thunderstorms are magnetic. We have solar fields, magnetic fields from electrical devices, motors, TVs, computers, wireless internet, wiring, and power lines, each producing subtle fields in the human body. Each can affect the magnetic energies in the body generated by cellular chemical reactions in the nervous system. Remember, increasing influxes of WiFi, GPS, and 5G can have a commutative effect on your nervous system and function.

There are toxins we cannot escape. But we can take measures and do the little things to reduce our exposure. We can also eat foods, supplement, breathe, and support our detoxification systems to help us live life and not live in fear. Toxic families, friends, and work have a negative impact on your digestion, immunity, blood sugar, and brain function. Find a way to spin the situation if you can't get out of it, or if you can, find a better environment more suited to your healthy life.

Once the human genome was sequenced, it was estimated that 90% of the human DNA was considered "junk." It's not important? If you look at the DNA in detail, it is a double helix, much the same as many galaxies of the cosmos. Why? Because it's stable. It contains an enormous amount of energy potential and a ridiculous amount of possibilities. Instead of this being considered "junk" by geneticists, it should be considered functional biomechanics with the possibility to function under all circumstances. It could be adjunct DNA aiding in the actions for the rest of the genome. That is, in fact, is what we are programmed to do. To be technical, a windshield or door was once considered junk to cars in their development state in the 1800s. But they're useful, convenient, and aid in safety. Without "junk," how else can we live in all places on Earth? How could we live under differing circumstances such as weather, sunlight, barometric pressure, temperature, food sources, and other environmental differences? It's because our DNA has the ability to adapt to individual stresses.

The good thing is we are surrounded by an abundance of energy. Some people don't see it, and I ask them to think of a soil and plant. All that's added over time is water. If you add up ten pounds of soil, a seed, and ten pounds water, then you should have twenty pounds in the end. But you don't. One may yield fifty pounds of plant. This doesn't add up. There's something else working. We know it's photosynthesis, and photosynthesis is energy from light. Thus, light is energy, energy is mass. And we know we are made from mass. And mass is from atoms, and only the nucleus is mass. In fact, it's rather logical when you think back to how we are made of atoms, and 99.9% of the atom is energy. Therefore, we are energy. As you can see, it's not that difficult to get here. Maybe it is a good idea to go for a walk on the beach. To play in the snow. To dig in the dirt. To not be isolated from the world. To breathe in nature and sit in the sun. Why? It is because they transfer energy, and that is what you are.

When you do little things to make you and your family healthy and when you get stuck, you combine what you were already doing with functional neurology/medicine/nutrition. Then integrate acupuncture, genetics, food plans, and exercise. Expect to get better.

When you get better, or at times worse, take no blame, take no credit. There's a much higher power at work, and you're a messenger. I bring the above up because you are now ready to help yourself, your family, and friends. The above statements combined with positive language and taking no credit means you can also take no blame. This will help keep you balanced in your mind and spirit so that you can be effective and protected.

Your body is designed to heal and be healthy through natural and normal reactions. When you sit back and think of all these reactions, it's quite a remarkable feat of intertwined communication. You are best in being a steward to the body, managing your energy through the mind and spirit. Each person is unique, and healing is an inside job. I believe anyone can do this and learn to influence the energies of their body to improve their health.

The ability to heal yourself is innate. It's of your ancestry and it resides within you, it's instinctual. Evolutionary psychologists have shown survival strategies in our DNA. Healing energies are embedded in your tissues, and you have healing abilities in your psyche. Our ancestors were able to hunt, build tools and shelters, and heal one another. Until the late 1800s, natural healing was the only option available. Our ancestors were only able to depend on themselves for their own survival, with no clinic and no antibiotics. They had to find food, herbs, and other treatments to regulate their energies and heal themselves. Humanity would not have survived the brutal and often hostile environments without this intuition. They figured out their basic needs of what was required to maintain life, and so will you.

RESOURCES

Acupuncture resources including acugraph

https://shortly.cc/k7MqF

Mash up program and autoimmunity education

https://shortly.cc/yB3uZ

Heart Rate Variability

https://shortly.cc/sjMsz

Emotional Freedom Technique

https://www.emofree.com/

Full Script Recommendations

marketing@newleafhealthandwellness.com

Brain Tap

https://shortly.cc/fhBjF

EMF reducer

shorturl.at/hTU59

Low light Laser Acupuncture and TeiShin

https://newleafhealthandwellness.com/shop/

Fast Mimicking Diet

Contact marketing@newleafhealthandwellness.com for the best discounted rate

Work out at home

https://8fit.com/dralantrites

Sauna

https://www.sunlighten.com

Recommendations from the book in sections below.

shorturl.at/syCU1

A. Brain- stimulation, balance, blue light blockers

B. Allergies

C. Air Purifiers and Dehumidifiers

D. Water Filters

E. Shower Filters

F. Nasal Help

G. Food Storage

H. Household Cleaners

I. Laundry

J. Weeding

K. Fertilizer

L. Body Wash

M. Deodorants

N. Hair Care

O. Creams

P. Sunscreens

Q. Toothpaste

R. Pulse Oximeter

Immune Points

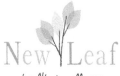

These points boost the immune system and should be rubbed for only 10 seconds two-three times each day. Do all points on both sides of your body for LU 1, LI 11 and LI 4.

Governing Vessel 20 (GV 20)—located at the top of the skull on the highest point of the head in the midline of the scalp

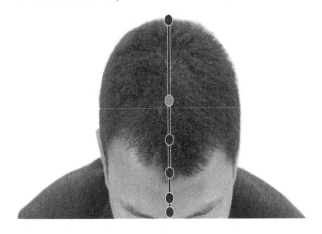

Cervical 7 (C7) & Thoracic 1 (T1)—this is the largest bump at the back of the neck

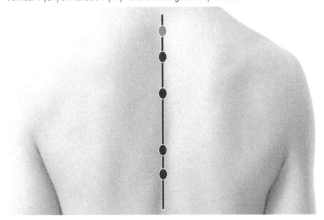

Lung 1 (LU 1)—on the outside of the chest in the first rib space, three inches from the midline and one-half inch below the clavicle

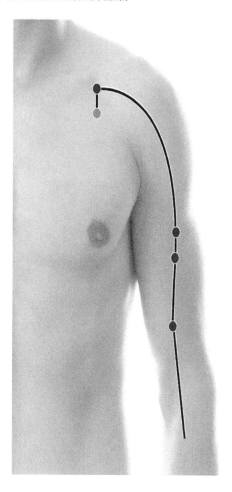

Thymus Point—but only do the right side, at the level of the thymus directly below the clavicle and two inches out from the sternum, only on the right side of the front

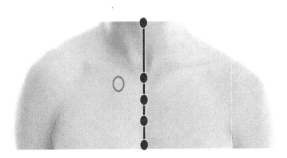

Lung 5 (LU 5)—at the elbow crease outside of the tendon connected to the bicep

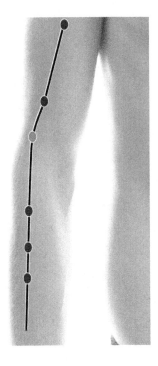

Large Intestine 11(LI 11) —located on the radial side of the elbow on the end of the outside elbow crease, when the forearm is flexed at a right angle too the upper arm

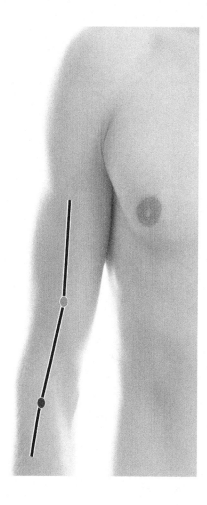

Large Intestine 4 (LI 4) —located in the thumb webbing between the thumb and the first finger, when the two digits are pushed together, where the crease ends is where the point remains

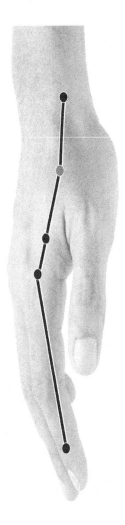

Stomach 35 (ST36) —if suffering from nausea or vomiting, add this point, located one finger length from the bone on the outside of the knee in the soft fleshy area between the kneecap and the outside bone (fibula)

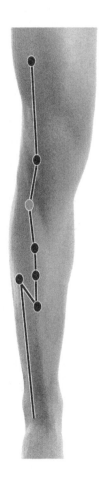

REFERENCES

Introduction

[1] "Computers versus Brains - Scientific American." 1 Nov. 2011, https://www.scientificamerican.com/article/computers-vs-brains/. Accessed 8 Jul. 2020.

[2] "Neuroscience For Kids - brain vs. computer." https://faculty.washington.edu/chudler/bvc.html. Accessed 8 Jul. 2020.

[3] "The Biochemical Origin of Pain: The origin of all Pain is ... - NCBI." https://www.ncbi.nlm.nih.gov/pmc/articles/PMC2771434/. Accessed 8 Jul. 2020.

[4] "The Neurobiology of Anxiety Disorders: Brain Imaging ...." https://www.ncbi.nlm.nih.gov/pmc/articles/PMC3684250/. Accessed 8 Jul. 2020.

[5] "Meridian Clock - Meridian Flow Wheel - Natural Health Zone." https://www.natural-health-zone.com/meridian-clock.html. Accessed 8 Jul. 2020.

[6] "Stress and Heart Rate Variability: A Meta-Analysis and ... - NCBI." 28 Feb. 2018, https://www.ncbi.nlm.nih.gov/pmc/articles/PMC5900369/. Accessed 8 Jul. 2020.

[7] "Measuring Overall Health System Performance for 191 ...." https://www.who.int/healthinfo/paper30.pdf?ua=1. Accessed 8 Jul. 2020.

[8] "Major Depression and Activation of the ... - PubMed." https://pubmed.ncbi.nlm.nih.gov/10442165/. Accessed 8 Jul. 2020.

[9] "Anatomy, Autonomic Nervous System - StatPearls - NCBI ...." 5 Apr. 2020, https://www.ncbi.nlm.nih.gov/books/NBK539845/. Accessed 8 Jul. 2020.

Chapter 1

[10] "Digitally numb: Doctors are losing hands-on diagnosis skills ...." 10 Jun. 2014, https://nationalpost.com/health/digitally-numb-doctors-are-losing-hands-on-diagnosis-skills-by-relying-too-much-on-technology. Accessed 8 Jul. 2020.

[11] "Commentary: Flow State (Trading the Sweat Spot for ... - NCBI." https://www.ncbi.nlm.nih.gov/pubmed/30239927. Accessed 8 Jul. 2020.

[12] "Obstetrical Malpractice Insurance - Medical Professional ...." https://www.ncbi.nlm.nih.gov/books/NBK218679/. Accessed 8 Jul. 2020.

[13] "FastStats - Therapeutic Drug Use - CDC." https://www.cdc.gov/nchs/fastats/drug-use-therapeutic.htm. Accessed 8 Jul. 2020.

[14] "Death by Medicine: Null, Gary, Feldman, Martin, Rasio ...." https://www.amazon.com/Death-Medicine-Gary-Null/dp/1607660067. Accessed 8 Jul. 2020.

[15] "Anatomy of an Epidemic: 9781491513217: Medicine & Health ...." https://www.amazon.com/Anatomy-Epidemic-Bullets-Psychiatric-Astonishing/dp/1491513217. Accessed 8 Jul. 2020.

[16] "Research into complementary and alternative medicine ...." https://www.ncbi.nlm.nih.gov/pmc/articles/PMC1119420/. Accessed 8 Jul. 2020.

[17] "Recommendations for Investigational COVID-19 ... - FDA." 1 May. 2020, https://www.fda.gov/vaccines-blood-biologics/investigational-new-drug-ind-or-device-exemption-ide-process-cber/recommendations-investigational-covid-19-convalescent-plasma. Accessed 8 Jul. 2020.

[18] "Convalescent Antibodies Infusion in COVID 19 Patients - Full ...." 5 Jun. 2020, https://clinicaltrials.gov/ct2/show/NCT04418531. Accessed 8 Jul. 2020.

[19] "Chronic Diseases in America | CDC." https://www.cdc.gov/chronicdisease/resources/infographic/chronic-diseases.htm. Accessed 8 Jul. 2020.

[20] "Annual Causes of Deaths in the United States." https://www.csdp.org/publicservice/causes.htm. Accessed 8 Jul. 2020.

[21] "Daily Aspirin Linked To More Than 3,000 Deaths Per Year ...." 14 Jun. 2017, https://www.huffingtonpost.co.uk/entry/daily-aspirin-causes-more-than-3000-deaths-per-year-scientists-warn_uk_593fb481e4b0b13f2c6daa10. Accessed 8 Jul. 2020.

[22] "Aspirin risk compares to driving cars, study finds - Reuters." 9 May. 2007, https://www.reuters.com/article/us-risks/aspirin-risk-compares-to-driving-cars-study-finds-idUSN0737156120070509. Accessed 8 Jul. 2020.

[23] "Acetaminophen: Avoiding Liver Injury | FDA." 24 Jun. 2009, https://www.fda.gov/consumers/consumer-updates/acetaminophen-avoiding-liver-injury. Accessed 8 Jul. 2020.

24 "Aspirin for Reducing Your Risk of Heart Attack and ... - FDA." 16 Dec. 2019, https://www.fda.gov/drugs/safe-daily-use-aspirin/aspirin-reducing-your-risk-heart-attack-and-stroke-know-facts. Accessed 8 Jul. 2020.

25 "Use of Aspirin for Primary Prevention of Heart Attack ... - FDA." 2 May. 2014, https://www.fda.gov/drugs/drug-information-consumers/use-aspirin-primary-prevention-heart-attack-and-stroke. Accessed 8 Jul. 2020.

26 "Can an Aspirin a Day Help Prevent a Heart Attack? | FDA." 5 May. 2014, https://www.fda.gov/consumers/consumer-updates/can-aspirin-day-help-prevent-heart-attack. Accessed 8 Jul. 2020.

27 "Before Using Aspirin to Lower Your Risk of Heart Attack ... - FDA." 22 Feb. 2016, https://www.fda.gov/drugs/safe-daily-use-aspirin/using-aspirin-lower-your-risk-heart-attack-or-stroke-what-you-should-know. Accessed 8 Jul. 2020.

28 "The Buying of the Congress: Charles Lewis: 9780380975969 ...." https://www.amazon.com/Buying-Congress-Charles-Lewis/dp/0380975963. Accessed 8 Jul. 2020.

29 "Most Experimental Drugs are Tested Offshore–Raising ...." 10 Sep. 2017, https://www.scientificamerican.com/article/most-experimental-drugs-are-tested-offshore-raising-concerns-about-data/. Accessed 8 Jul. 2020.

30 "Drug Quality Sampling and Testing Programs | FDA." 3 Feb. 2020, https://www.fda.gov/drugs/science-and-research-drugs/drug-quality-sampling-and-testing-programs. Accessed 8 Jul. 2020.

[31] "U.S. Dependence on Pharmaceutical Products From China ...." 14 Aug. 2019, https://www.cfr.org/blog/us-dependence-pharmaceutical-products-china. Accessed 8 Jul. 2020.

[32] "Medical errors third-leading cause of death in America." 22 Feb. 2018, https://www.cnbc.com/2018/02/22/medical-errors-third-leading-cause-of-death-in-america.html. Accessed 8 Jul. 2020.

[33] "FastStats - Accidents or Unintentional Injuries - CDC." https://www.cdc.gov/nchs/fastats/accidental-injury.htm. Accessed 8 Jul. 2020.

[34] "Key Data and Statistics|WISQARS|Injury Center|CDC." https://www.cdc.gov/injury/wisqars/overview/key_data.html. Accessed 8 Jul. 2020.

Chapter 2

[35] "What is Functional Medicine? | IFM." https://www.ifm.org/functional-medicine/what-is-functional-medicine/. Accessed 8 Jul. 2020.

[36] "American College of Functional Neurology – Credentialing ...." https://acfn.org/. Accessed 8 Jul. 2020.

[37] "Neuroplasticity and Clinical Practice: Building Brain Power for ...." 26 Jul. 2016, https://www.ncbi.nlm.nih.gov/pmc/articles/PMC4960264/. Accessed 8 Jul. 2020.

[38] "Aging and neuroplasticity - NCBI." https://www.ncbi.nlm.nih.gov/pmc/articles/PMC3622467/. Accessed 8 Jul. 2020.

[39] "Brain Plasticity and Behaviour in the Developing Brain - NCBI." https://www.ncbi.nlm.nih.gov/pmc/articles/PMC3222570/. Accessed 8 Jul. 2020.

[40] "Magnetic Resonance, Functional (fMRI) - Brain." https://www.radiologyinfo.org/en/info.cfm?pg=fmribrain. Accessed 8 Jul. 2020.

[41] "Placebos and Blinding in Randomized Controlled ... - FDA." 23 Oct. 2019, https://www.fda.gov/regulatory-information/search-fda-guidance-documents/placebos-and-blinding-randomized-controlled-cancer-clinical-trials-drug-and-biological-products. Accessed 8 Jul. 2020.

[42] "Guidance for Industry - FDA." https://www.fda.gov/media/71349/download. Accessed 8 Jul. 2020.

[43] "FDA and Clinical Drug Trials: A Short History." https://www.fda.gov/media/110437/download. Accessed 8 Jul. 2020.

[44] "Psychoneuroimmunology: Definition, Research, and Examples." 26 Jan. 2018, https://www.healthline.com/health/psychoneuroimmunology. Accessed 8 Jul. 2020.

Chapter 3

[45] "Top tips to deal with challenging situations: doctor–patient ...." https://www.ncbi.nlm.nih.gov/pmc/articles/PMC5467659/. Accessed 8 Jul. 2020.

[46] "Applications of Mass Spectrometry for Cellular Lipid Analysis." 19 Jan. 2015, https://www.ncbi.nlm.nih.gov/pmc/articles/PMC4376555/. Accessed 8 Jul. 2020.

47 "Health Care Spending in US, Other High-Income Countries." 13 Mar. 2018, https://www.commonwealthfund.org/publications/journal-article/2018/mar/health-care-spending-united-states-and-other-high-income. Accessed 8 Jul. 2020.

48 "U.S. health expenditure as percent of GDP 1960-2020 - Statista." 8 Jun. 2020, https://www.statista.com/statistics/184968/us-health-expenditure-as-percent-of-gdp-since-1960/. Accessed 8 Jul. 2020.

49 "Only 23% of Americans Get Enough Exercise, a CDC Report ...." 28 Jun. 2018, https://time.com/5324940/americans-exercise-physical-activity-guidelines/. Accessed 8 Jul. 2020.

50 "CDC: 80 percent of American adults don't get recommended ...." 3 May. 2013, https://www.cbsnews.com/news/cdc-80-percent-of-american-adults-dont-get-recommended-exercise/. Accessed 8 Jul. 2020.

51 "Physical Activity Guidelines for Americans | HHS.gov." https://www.hhs.gov/fitness/be-active/physical-activity-guidelines-for-americans/index.html. Accessed 8 Jul. 2020.

Chapter 4

52 "Insurers restricting choice of doctors and hospitals to keep ...." 20 Nov. 2013, https://www.washingtonpost.com/national/health-science/insurers-restricting-choice-of-doctors-and-hospitals-to-keep-costs-down/2013/11/20/98c84e20-4bb4-11e3-ac54-aa84301ced81_story.html. Accessed 8 Jul. 2020.

53 "Risk of thyroid cancer based on thyroid ultrasound findings." https://www.thyroid.org/patient-thyroid-information/ct-for-patients/vol-7-issue-1/vol-7-issue-1-p-6-7/. Accessed 8 Jul. 2020.

[54] "Calculate Your BMI - Standard BMI Calculator - NIH." https://www.nhlbi.nih.gov/health/educational/lose_wt/BMI/bmicalc.htm. Accessed 8 Jul. 2020.

[55] "Adult BMI Calculator | Healthy Weight | CDC." 6 Jul. 2020, https://www.cdc.gov/healthyweight/assessing/bmi/adult_bmi/english_bmi_calculator/bmi_calculator.html. Accessed 8 Jul. 2020.

[56] "DWI Detection and Standardized Field Sobriety Test ... - NHTSA." https://www.nhtsa.gov/sites/nhtsa.dot.gov/files/documents/sfst_ig_refresher_manual.pdf. Accessed 8 Jul. 2020.

[57] "Sporadic Cerebellar Ataxia Associated With Gluten Sensitivity." https://pubmed.ncbi.nlm.nih.gov/11335703/. Accessed 8 Jul. 2020.

[58] "Cerebellar Ataxia, Celiac Disease and Non-Celiac Gluten ...." https://sites.kowsarpub.com/ans/articles/14280.html. Accessed 8 Jul. 2020.

[59] "Sporadic cerebellar ataxia associated with gluten sensitivity ...." https://academic.oup.com/brain/article/124/5/1013/309958. Accessed 8 Jul. 2020.

[60] "Dietary treatment of gluten ataxia | Journal of Neurology ...." https://jnnp.bmj.com/content/74/9/1221. Accessed 8 Jul. 2020.

[61] "Cerebellar Disorders due to Gluten sensitivity - Dizziness-and ...." 15 Jul. 2019, https://www.dizziness-and-balance.com/disorders/central/cerebellar/gluten.htm. Accessed 8 Jul. 2020.

[62] "Motor Phenotype in Neurodegenerative Disorders: Gait ... - NCBI." 17 Jul. 2017, https://www.ncbi.nlm.nih.gov/pmc/articles/PMC5523841/. Accessed 8 Jul. 2020.

[63] "Motor Phenotype in Neurodegenerative Disorders: Gait and ...." https://pubmed.ncbi.nlm.nih.gov/28671116/. Accessed 8 Jul. 2020.

[64] "Laboratory Medicine Curriculum - WebPath." https://webpath.med.utah.edu/EXAM/LabMedCurric/LabMed01_02.html. Accessed 8 Jul. 2020.

[65] "Learn how reference range is determined for laboratory tests." http://www.clinlabnavigator.com/reference-ranges.html. Accessed 8 Jul. 2020.

Chapter 5

[66] "Microscopes and accessories - FDA." https://www.accessdata.fda.gov/scripts/cdrh/cfdocs/cfcfr/CFRSearch.cfm?fr=864.3600. Accessed 8 Jul. 2020.

[67] "CPG Sec. 370.100 Cytotoxic Testing for Allergic Diseases | FDA." 24 Sep. 1987, https://www.fda.gov/regulatory-information/search-fda-guidance-documents/cpg-sec-370100-cytotoxic-testing-allergic-diseases. Accessed 8 Jul. 2020.

[68] "Use of International Standard ISO 10993-1, "Biological ... - FDA." 16 Jun. 2016, https://www.fda.gov/media/85865/download. Accessed 8 Jul. 2020.

[69] "Costs of Alzheimer's to Medicare and Medicaid." https://act.alz.org/site/DocServer/2012_Costs_Fact_Sheet_version_2.pdf?docID=7161. Accessed 8 Jul. 2020.

[70] "Elevated Basal Cortisol Level Predicts Lower Hippocampal ...." https://pubmed.ncbi.nlm.nih.gov/19570680/. Accessed 10 Jul. 2020.

[71] "Homocysteine and Brain Atrophy on MRI of Non ... - PubMed." https://pubmed.ncbi.nlm.nih.gov/12477704/. Accessed 10 Jul. 2020.

[72] "Reactive oxygen species stimulate central and peripheral ...." https://www.ncbi.nlm.nih.gov/pubmed/15277201. Accessed 10 Jul. 2020.

[73] "Changes in enzymatic antioxidant defense system in blood ...." https://www.ncbi.nlm.nih.gov/pubmed/9507566. Accessed 10 Jul. 2020.

[74] "Cognitive Improvement in Mild to Moderate Alzheimer's ...." https://pubmed.ncbi.nlm.nih.gov/12637119/. Accessed 10 Jul. 2020.

[75] "Huperzine A for Alzheimer's Disease - PubMed." 16 Apr. 2008, https://pubmed.ncbi.nlm.nih.gov/18425924/. Accessed 10 Jul. 2020.

[76] "Long-term acetyl-L-carnitine Treatment in Alzheimer's Disease." https://pubmed.ncbi.nlm.nih.gov/1944900. Accessed 10 Jul. 2020.

[77] "Testosterone Reduces Neuronal Secretion of Alzheimer's ...." 1 Feb. 2000, https://pubmed.ncbi.nlm.nih.gov/10655508/. Accessed 10 Jul. 2020.

[78] "Apolipoprotein E and Alzheimer Disease: Risk, Mechanisms ...." 8 Jan. 2013, https://pubmed.ncbi.nlm.nih.gov/23296339/. Accessed 10 Jul. 2020.

[79] "Association of Coffee and Caffeine Intake With the Risk of ...." https://pubmed.ncbi.nlm.nih.gov/10819950/. Accessed 10 Jul. 2020.

[80] "Mental Training for Cognitive Improvement in Elderly People ...." https://pubmed.ncbi.nlm.nih.gov/26238812. Accessed 10 Jul. 2020.

[81] "A review on the acute phase response in major depression.." https://www.ncbi.nlm.nih.gov/pubmed/7506108. Accessed 8 Jul. 2020.

[82] "Neurodegeneration: a key factor in the ageing gut. - NCBI." https://www.ncbi.nlm.nih.gov/pubmed/15065999. Accessed 8 Jul. 2020.

[83] "The Gut-Brain Barrier in Major Depression: Intestinal Mucosal ...." https://pubmed.ncbi.nlm.nih.gov/18283240. Accessed 8 Jul. 2020.

[84] "Potential role of cerebral glutathione in the maintenance of ...." https://www.ncbi.nlm.nih.gov/pubmed/10591399. Accessed 8 Jul. 2020.

[85] "Structural and functional adaptation to hypoxia in the rat brain.." https://pubmed.ncbi.nlm.nih.gov/15299038/. Accessed 8 Jul. 2020.

[86] "Age-related changes of the nitric oxide system in the rat brain.." https://www.ncbi.nlm.nih.gov/pubmed/12445710. Accessed 8 Jul. 2020.

[87] "Roles of nitric oxide in brain hypoxia-ischemia. - NCBI." https://www.ncbi.nlm.nih.gov/pubmed/10320673. Accessed 8 Jul. 2020.

[88] "Excitatory Amino Acid Neurotoxicity - Madame Curie ... - NCBI." https://www.ncbi.nlm.nih.gov/books/NBK6108/. Accessed 8 Jul. 2020.

[89] "Excitatory Amino Acids as a Final Common Pathway for ...." 3 Mar. 1994, https://www.nejm.org/doi/10.1056/ NEJM199403033300907. Accessed 8 Jul. 2020.

[90] "Deciphering the MSG controversy - NCBI." 15 Nov. 2009, https://www.ncbi.nlm.nih.gov/pmc/articles/PMC2802046/. Accessed 8 Jul. 2020.

[91] "Heavy NSAID Use Linked to Higher Dementia Risk | MedPage ...." 22 Apr. 2009, https://www.medpagetoday.org/psychiatry/alzheimersdisease/13860. Accessed 8 Jul. 2020.

[92] "Risk of dementia and AD with prior exposure to NSAIDs in an ...." 22 Apr. 2009, https://www.ncbi.nlm.nih.gov/pubmed/19386997. Accessed 8 Jul. 2020.

[93] "High Fructose Corn Syrup and the Brain - David Perlmutter M.D.." 9 Feb. 2016, https://www.drperlmutter.com/high-fructose-corn-syrup-brain/. Accessed 8 Jul. 2020.

[94] "The emerging role of dietary fructose in obesity and cognitive ...." 8 Aug. 2013, https://www.ncbi.nlm.nih.gov/pmc/articles/PMC3751294/. Accessed 8 Jul. 2020.

[95] "Elevated cortisol in older adults with Generalized Anxiety ...." https://www.ncbi.nlm.nih.gov/pmc/articles/PMC3424606/. Accessed 8 Jul. 2020.

[96] "Cortisol Secretion in Depressed and At-Risk Adults - NCBI." 2 Nov. 2012, https://www.ncbi.nlm.nih.gov/pmc/articles/PMC4451064/. Accessed 8 Jul. 2020.

[97] "Estrogen, Cytokines, and Pathogenesis of Postmenopausal ...." https://pubmed.ncbi.nlm.nih.gov/8854239/. Accessed 8 Jul. 2020.

[98] "Oestradiol decreases colonic permeability through oestrogen ...." 11 May. 2009, https://www.ncbi.nlm.nih.gov/pmc/articles/PMC2727039/. Accessed 8 Jul. 2020.

[99] "Leptin resistance: underlying mechanisms and diagnosis - NCBI." 25 Jan. 2019, https://www.ncbi.nlm.nih.gov/pmc/articles/PMC6354688/. Accessed 8 Jul. 2020.

[100] "Role of C-Reactive Protein at Sites of Inflammation and Infection." 13 Apr. 2018, https://www.ncbi.nlm.nih.gov/pmc/articles/PMC5908901/. Accessed 8 Jul. 2020.

[101] "The crucial role of metal ions in neurodegeneration: the basis ...." 3 Oct. 2005, https://www.ncbi.nlm.nih.gov/pmc/articles/PMC1751240/. Accessed 8 Jul. 2020.

[102] "Neuroantibody Biomarkers: Links and Challenges in ... - NCBI." 23 Jun. 2014, https://www.ncbi.nlm.nih.gov/pmc/articles/PMC4090524/. Accessed 8 Jul. 2020.

[103] "Electromagnetic fields and public health - WHO." https://www.who.int/peh-emf/publications/facts/fs296/en/. Accessed 8 Jul. 2020.

[104] "Thyroid hormone induces protein secretion and morphological ...." https://www.ncbi.nlm.nih.gov/pubmed/9246951. Accessed 8 Jul. 2020.

[105] "Microglia: Intrinsic Immuneffector Cell of the Brain - PubMed." https://pubmed.ncbi.nlm.nih.gov/7550361/. Accessed 8 Jul. 2020.

[106] "National Toxicology Program (NTP) Division." https://www.niehs.nih.gov/research/atniehs/dntp/index.cfm. Accessed 8 Jul. 2020.

[107] "Childhood Lead Exposure and Adult Neurodegenerative ...." https://www.ncbi.nlm.nih.gov/pmc/articles/PMC6454899/. Accessed 8 Jul. 2020.

[108] "Is aluminum exposure a risk factor for neurological disorders?."
6 Jun. 2018, https://www.ncbi.nlm.nih.gov/pmc/articles/
PMC6040147/. Accessed 8 Jul. 2020.

[109] "DHA Effects in Brain Development and Function - NCBI."
https://www.ncbi.nlm.nih.gov/pmc/articles/PMC4728620/.
Accessed 10 Jul. 2020.

[110] "Role of docosahexaenoic acid in maternal and child mental ...."
28 Jan. 2009, https://academic.oup.com/ajcn/article-abstract/
89/3/958S/4596814. Accessed 10 Jul. 2020.

[111] "Effect of docosahexaenoic acid-fortified Chlorella vulgaris ...."
https://www.ncbi.nlm.nih.gov/pubmed/12186415. Accessed 8 Jul.
2020.

[112] "Chronic administration of docosahexaenoic acid improves ...."
https://www.ncbi.nlm.nih.gov/pubmed/10430487. Accessed 8 Jul.
2020.

[113] "The effect of 17beta-estradiol on production of cytokines in ...."
https://www.ncbi.nlm.nih.gov/pubmed/11472888. Accessed 8 Jul.
2020.

[114] "Essential fatty acids preparation (SR-3) improves
Alzheimer's ...." https://www.ncbi.nlm.nih.gov/pubmed/9003975.
Accessed 8 Jul. 2020.

[115] "Effects of antioxidant supplementation and exercise
training ...." https://www.ncbi.nlm.nih.gov/pubmed/17245671.
Accessed 8 Jul. 2020.

116 "Neurofeedback: A Comprehensive Review on System Design ...." https://www.ncbi.nlm.nih.gov/pmc/articles/PMC4892319/. Accessed 8 Jul. 2020.

117 "Glyphosate weed killers increase cancer risk by 41%, study says." 15 Feb. 2019, https://www.cnn.com/2019/02/14/health/us-glyphosate-cancer-study-scli-intl/index.html. Accessed 8 Jul. 2020.

118 "UW study: Exposure to chemical in Roundup increases risk for ...." 13 Feb. 2019, https://www.washington.edu/news/2019/02/13/uw-study-exposure-to-chemical-in-roundup-increases-risk-for-cancer/. Accessed 8 Jul. 2020.

119 "Review of the neurological benefits of phytocannabinoids - NCBI." 26 Apr. 2018, https://www.ncbi.nlm.nih.gov/pmc/articles/PMC5938896/. Accessed 8 Jul. 2020.

120 "CBD vs. THC: Properties, Benefits, and Side Effects - Healthline." https://www.healthline.com/health/cbd-vs-thc. Accessed 8 Jul. 2020.

121 "Sympathovagal Balance: How Should We ...." https://pubmed.ncbi.nlm.nih.gov/10199852/. Accessed 10 Jul. 2020.

122 "Saccade and vestibular ocular motor adaptation. - NCBI - NIH." https://www.ncbi.nlm.nih.gov/pubmed/20086279. Accessed 10 Jul. 2020.

123 "Effects of blue light on the circadian system and eye physiology." 24 Jan. 2016, https://www.ncbi.nlm.nih.gov/pmc/articles/PMC4734149/. Accessed 10 Jul. 2020.

[124] "Physical and Immunological Aspects of Exercise in Chronic ...." https://pubmed.ncbi.nlm.nih.gov/25428651/. Accessed 10 Jul. 2020.

[125] "Memory-guided microsaccades | Nature Communications." 16 Aug. 2019, https://www.nature.com/articles/s41467-019-11711-x. Accessed 10 Jul. 2020.

[126] "Why Is Synaptic Pruning Important for the Developing Brain ...." 1 May. 2017, https://www.scientificamerican.com/article/why-is-synaptic-pruning-important-for-the-developing-brain/. Accessed 8 Jul. 2020.

[127] "Inflammation and Immune Function - Antioxidants in Sport ...." https://www.ncbi.nlm.nih.gov/books/NBK299041/. Accessed 8 Jul. 2020.

Chapter 6

[128] "Prevalence and Sociodemographic Correlates of Antinuclear ...." https://www.ncbi.nlm.nih.gov/pmc/articles/PMC3330150/. Accessed 8 Jul. 2020.

[129] "Sodium chloride drives autoimmune disease by the induction ...." 6 Mar. 2013, https://www.nature.com/articles/nature11868. Accessed 8 Jul. 2020.

[130] "The impact of wavelengths of LED light-therapy on endothelial ...." 6 Sep. 2017, https://www.nature.com/articles/s41598-017-11061-y. Accessed 8 Jul. 2020.

[131] "Effects of caffeine on sleep quality and daytime functioning." 7 Dec. 2018, https://www.ncbi.nlm.nih.gov/pmc/articles/PMC6292246/. Accessed 8 Jul. 2020.

132 "Prevalence of Thyroid Antibodies Among Healthy Middle ...." https://pubmed.ncbi.nlm.nih.gov/7606312/. Accessed 8 Jul. 2020.

133 "Nocturnal Hypoglycemia Identified by a Continuous Glucose ...." https://www.ncbi.nlm.nih.gov/pmc/articles/PMC3338953/. Accessed 8 Jul. 2020.

134 "Aerobic Exercise Improves Hippocampal Function ... - PubMed." https://pubmed.ncbi.nlm.nih.gov/21722657/. Accessed 10 Jul. 2020.

135 "Daily timing of salivary cortisol responses and aerobic ... - NCBI." https://www.ncbi.nlm.nih.gov/pubmed/21585131. Accessed 10 Jul. 2020.

136 "Heart Rate Variability to Assess the Changes in Autonomic ...." 13 Oct. 2017, https://www.researchgate.net/publication/320306138_Heart_Rate_Variability_to_Assess_the_Changes_in_Autonomic_Nervous_System_Function_Associated_With_Vertebral_Subluxation. Accessed 10 Jul. 2020.

137 "Heart Rate Variability to Assess the Changes in Autonomic ...." 13 Oct. 2017, https://www.researchgate.net/publication/320306138_Heart_Rate_Variability_to_Assess_the_Changes_in_Autonomic_Nervous_System_Function_Associated_With_Vertebral_Subluxation. Accessed 10 Jul. 2020.

138 "Determinants of Heart Rate Variability - PubMed." https://pubmed.ncbi.nlm.nih.gov/8917269/. Accessed 10 Jul. 2020.

139 "The role of heart rate variability in sports physiology - NCBI." 23 Feb. 2016, https://www.ncbi.nlm.nih.gov/pmc/articles/PMC4840584/. Accessed 10 Jul. 2020.

[140] "Effect of Endurance Exercise Training on Heart Rate ...." https://pubmed.ncbi.nlm.nih.gov/9832101/. Accessed 10 Jul. 2020.

[141] "Heart Rate Variability: Standards of Measurement, Physiological." https://pubmed.ncbi.nlm.nih.gov/8598068/. Accessed 10 Jul. 2020.

[142] "Cardiac arrest caused by trigeminal neuralgia. - NCBI." https://www.ncbi.nlm.nih.gov/pubmed/8707560. Accessed 10 Jul. 2020.

[143] "The "straight back" syndrome: current perspective more ... - NCBI." https://www.ncbi.nlm.nih.gov/pubmed/3995803. Accessed 10 Jul. 2020.

[144] "The application of neurologic reflexes to the treatment ... - NCBI." https://www.ncbi.nlm.nih.gov/pubmed/583146. Accessed 10 Jul. 2020.

[145] "New method for assessing cardiac parasympathetic activity ...." https://www.ncbi.nlm.nih.gov/pubmed/6383446. Accessed 10 Jul. 2020.

[146] "Glutathione peroxidase 1 deficiency attenuates allergen ...." 1 Sep. 2010, https://www.ncbi.nlm.nih.gov/pubmed/20367278. Accessed 8 Jul. 2020.

[147] "Glutathione catabolism as a signaling mechanism. - NCBI." https://www.ncbi.nlm.nih.gov/pubmed/12213602. Accessed 8 Jul. 2020.

[148] "Oxidative stress and enhanced paracellular permeability in ...." 16 Sep. 2009, https://www.ncbi.nlm.nih.gov/pubmed/19756603. Accessed 8 Jul. 2020.

[149] "Glutathione depletion upregulates P-glycoprotein expression ...." https://www.ncbi.nlm.nih.gov/pubmed/19505374. Accessed 8 Jul. 2020.

[150] "Potential role of cerebral glutathione in the maintenance of ...." https://www.ncbi.nlm.nih.gov/pubmed/10591399. Accessed 8 Jul. 2020.

[151] "Glutathione Dysregulation and the Etiology and Progression ...." https://pubmed.ncbi.nlm.nih.gov/19166318/. Accessed 8 Jul. 2020.

[152] "Age-related changes in glutathione and ... - NCBI - NIH." https://www.ncbi.nlm.nih.gov/pubmed/16647047. Accessed 8 Jul. 2020.

[153] "Selenium, glutathione peroxidase (GSH-Px) and lipid ...." 30 Apr. 1992, https://www.sciencedirect.com/science/article/pii/000989819290157L. Accessed 8 Jul. 2020.

[154] "GPR109a: The Missing Link between Microbiome and Good ...." https://www.ncbi.nlm.nih.gov/pmc/articles/PMC4337780/. Accessed 8 Jul. 2020.

[155] "Gut Microbiome as Target for Innovative Strategies Against ...." 15 Feb. 2019, https://www.ncbi.nlm.nih.gov/pmc/articles/PMC6384262/. Accessed 8 Jul. 2020.

[156] "Gut Microbiome as Target for Innovative Strategies Against ...." 15 Feb. 2019, https://www.ncbi.nlm.nih.gov/pmc/articles/PMC6384262/. Accessed 8 Jul. 2020.

157 "A Study in Balance: How Microbiomes Are Changing the ...." 1 Aug. 2011, https://www.ncbi.nlm.nih.gov/pmc/articles/ PMC3237378/. Accessed 8 Jul. 2020.

158 "Curcumin: A Review of Its' Effects on Human Health - NCBI." 22 Oct. 2017, https://www.ncbi.nlm.nih.gov/pmc/articles/ PMC5664031/. Accessed 8 Jul. 2020.

159 "Mitochondrial decay in the brains of old rats: ameliorating ...." 10 Oct. 2019, https://www.ncbi.nlm.nih.gov/pubmed/18846423. Accessed 8 Jul. 2020.

160 "Regulatory role of resveratrol on Th17 in autoimmune disease.." https://www.ncbi.nlm.nih.gov/pubmed/20708723. Accessed 8 Jul. 2020.

161 "Epidemiology of Vitamin D in Health and Disease - PubMed." https://pubmed.ncbi.nlm.nih.gov/19860998/. Accessed 8 Jul. 2020.

162 "Vitamin D and the Immune System - NCBI - NIH." 1 Aug. 2012, https://www.ncbi.nlm.nih.gov/pmc/articles/PMC3166406/. Accessed 8 Jul. 2020.

163 "Epidemic Influenza and Vitamin D - PubMed." https:// pubmed.ncbi.nlm.nih.gov/16959053/. Accessed 8 Jul. 2020.

164 "On the epidemiology of influenza | Virology Journal | Full Text." 25 Feb. 2008, https://virologyj.biomedcentral.com/articles/ 10.1186/1743-422X-5-29. Accessed 8 Jul. 2020.

165 "Vitamin K-dependent gamma-carboxylation of the 1,25 ...." https://www.ncbi.nlm.nih.gov/pubmed/1336373. Accessed 8 Jul. 2020.

166 "Study of the nitric oxide system in the rat cerebellum during ...." 24 Jun. 2010, https://www.ncbi.nlm.nih.gov/pubmed/ 20576087. Accessed 8 Jul. 2020.

167 "Erectile Dysfunction and L-Citrulline: What You Should Know." https://www.healthline.com/health/erectile-dysfunction/l-citrulline. Accessed 8 Jul. 2020.

168 "Supplemental Citrulline Is More Efficient Than Arginine in ...." 8 Feb. 2017, https://www.ncbi.nlm.nih.gov/pmc/articles/ PMC5368575/. Accessed 8 Jul. 2020.

169 "Hepcidin and iron regulation, 10 years later - NCBI." https:// www.ncbi.nlm.nih.gov/pmc/articles/PMC3099567/. Accessed 8 Jul. 2020.

170 "An update on Vinpocetine: New discoveries and clinical ...." https://www.ncbi.nlm.nih.gov/pmc/articles/PMC5766389/. Accessed 8 Jul. 2020.

171 "ProLon Fasting Mimicking Diet Review: Does It Work for ...." 29 Jan. 2019, https://www.healthline.com/nutrition/fasting-mimicking-diet. Accessed 8 Jul. 2020.

172 "Gymnema sylvestre: A Memoir - NCBI." 29 Aug. 2007, https:// www.ncbi.nlm.nih.gov/pmc/articles/PMC2170951/. Accessed 8 Jul. 2020.

173 "Vanadium and Diabetes - PubMed." https:// pubmed.ncbi.nlm.nih.gov/9823013/. Accessed 8 Jul. 2020.

174 "A Scientific Review: The Role of Chromium in Insulin Resistance." https://pubmed.ncbi.nlm.nih.gov/15208835/. Accessed 8 Jul. 2020.

[175] "Human Zonulin, a Potential Modulator of Intestinal Tight ...." https://pubmed.ncbi.nlm.nih.gov/11082037. Accessed 8 Jul. 2020.

[176] "IL-1β-Induced Increase in Intestinal Epithelial Tight Junction ...." https://www.ncbi.nlm.nih.gov/pmc/articles/PMC2966790/. Accessed 8 Jul. 2020.

[177] "Tight junctions, leaky intestines, and pediatric diseases ...." https://www.ncbi.nlm.nih.gov/pubmed/16092447/. Accessed 8 Jul. 2020.

[178] "Human Zonulin, a Potential Modulator of Intestinal Tight ...." https://pubmed.ncbi.nlm.nih.gov/11082037. Accessed 8 Jul. 2020.

[179] "Can Allergy Medications Harm Your Brain? | Cognitive Vitality ...." 25 Apr. 2018, https://www.alzdiscovery.org/cognitive-vitality/blog/can-allergy-medications-harm-your-brain. Accessed 8 Jul. 2020.

[180] "Common anticholinergic drugs like Benadryl linked to ...." 25 Jun. 2019, https://www.health.harvard.edu/blog/common-anticholinergic-drugs-like-benadryl-linked-increased-dementia-risk-201501287667. Accessed 8 Jul. 2020.

[181] "Long-term Anti-inflammatory and Antihistamine Medication ...." https://www.ncbi.nlm.nih.gov/pmc/articles/PMC6436627/. Accessed 8 Jul. 2020.

[182] "Zinc in Human Health: Effect of Zinc on Immune Cells." 3 Apr. 2008, https://www.ncbi.nlm.nih.gov/pmc/articles/PMC2277319/. Accessed 8 Jul. 2020.

[183] "Possible Roles of Magnesium on the Immune System - PubMed." https://pubmed.ncbi.nlm.nih.gov/14506478/. Accessed 8 Jul. 2020.

Chapter 7

[184] "Autoimmune Statistics — The Autoimmune Registry." https://www.autoimmuneregistry.org/autoimmune-statistics. Accessed 8 Jul. 2020.

[185] "Autoimmunity: basic mechanisms and implications in ... - NCBI." https://www.ncbi.nlm.nih.gov/pubmed/16807508. Accessed 8 Jul. 2020.

[186] "The Gluten Syndrome: A Neurological Disease - PubMed." 29 Apr. 2009, https://pubmed.ncbi.nlm.nih.gov/19406584. Accessed 10 Jul. 2020.

[187] "The gluten syndrome: A neurological disease - Dr. Perlmutter." http://www.drperlmutter.com/wp-content/uploads/2013/07/17-The_gluten_syndrome__A_neurological_disease1.pdf. Accessed 10 Jul. 2020.

[188] "Elevated levels of antibodies against xenobiotics in a ... - NCBI." 18 Jul. 2014, https://www.ncbi.nlm.nih.gov/pmc/articles/PMC4365752/. Accessed 8 Jul. 2020.

[189] "Diagnostic Testing and Interpretation of Tests for Autoimmunity." 12 Jan. 2010, https://www.ncbi.nlm.nih.gov/pmc/articles/PMC2832720/. Accessed 8 Jul. 2020.

[190] "Risk Factors for and Prevalence of Thyroid Disorders in a Cross." https://pubmed.ncbi.nlm.nih.gov/12919165. Accessed 8 Jul. 2020.

[191] "Risk of Subclinical Hypothyroidism in Pregnant Women With ...." https://pubmed.ncbi.nlm.nih.gov/8027226/. Accessed 8 Jul. 2020.

[192] "[Thyroid function and thyroid autoimmunity at the late ... - NCBI." https://www.ncbi.nlm.nih.gov/pubmed/17083836. Accessed 8 Jul. 2020.

[193] "Host-dependent Zonulin Secretion Causes the Impairment of ...." https://pubmed.ncbi.nlm.nih.gov/12404235/. Accessed 10 Jul. 2020.

[194] "Host-dependent Zonulin Secretion Causes the Impairment of ...." https://pubmed.ncbi.nlm.nih.gov/12404235/. Accessed 10 Jul. 2020.

[195] "Receptor for Advanced Glycation Endproducts Mediates ...." 15 Feb. 2007, https://www.jimmunol.org/content/178/4/2483. Accessed 10 Jul. 2020.

[196] "Receptor for Advanced Glycation Endproducts Mediates ...." https://pubmed.ncbi.nlm.nih.gov/17277156/. Accessed 10 Jul. 2020.

[197] "The Gut-Brain Barrier in Major Depression: Intestinal Mucosal ...." https://pubmed.ncbi.nlm.nih.gov/18283240. Accessed 10 Jul. 2020.

[198] "Comparison of Bruker Biotyper matrix-assisted laser ... - NCBI." 5 Jan. 2011, https://www.ncbi.nlm.nih.gov/pubmed/21209160. Accessed 10 Jul. 2020.

[199] "The Prevalence of Antibodies against Wheat and Milk Proteins ...." 19 Dec. 2013, https://www.ncbi.nlm.nih.gov/pmc/articles/PMC3916846/. Accessed 10 Jul. 2020.

[200] "Migration and proliferation of mononuclear phagocytes ... - NCBI." https://www.ncbi.nlm.nih.gov/pubmed/9413568. Accessed 10 Jul. 2020.

[201] "Zonulin and Its Regulation of Intestinal Barrier Function: The ...." https://pubmed.ncbi.nlm.nih.gov/21248165/. Accessed 10 Jul. 2020.

[202] "Levels of vasoactive intestinal peptide, cholecystokinin ... - NCBI." https://www.ncbi.nlm.nih.gov/pmc/articles/PMC4727008/. Accessed 10 Jul. 2020.

[203] "Intestinal permeability – a new target for disease prevention ...." 18 Nov. 2014, https://www.ncbi.nlm.nih.gov/pmc/articles/PMC4253991/. Accessed 8 Jul. 2020.

[204] "Alterations in intestinal permeability - NCBI." https://www.ncbi.nlm.nih.gov/pmc/articles/PMC1856434/. Accessed 8 Jul. 2020.

[205] "Artificial intelligence in clinical and genomic diagnostics ...." 19 Nov. 2019, https://genomemedicine.biomedcentral.com/articles/10.1186/s13073-019-0689-8. Accessed 8 Jul. 2020.

[206] "Mechanisms of human autoimmunity - JCI." 20 Apr. 2015, https://www.jci.org/articles/view/78088/figure/1. Accessed 8 Jul. 2020.

[207] "Myopathy Associated With Gluten Sensitivity - PubMed." https://pubmed.ncbi.nlm.nih.gov/17143894. Accessed 8 Jul. 2020.

[208] "Sensory Ganglionopathy Due to Gluten Sensitivity - PubMed." 14 Sep. 2010, https://pubmed.ncbi.nlm.nih.gov/20837968/. Accessed 8 Jul. 2020.

[209] "Headache and CNS White Matter Abnormalities Associated ...." https://pubmed.ncbi.nlm.nih.gov/11171906/. Accessed 8 Jul. 2020.

[210] "Recent advances in understanding non-celiac gluten sensitivity." 11 Oct. 2018, https://www.ncbi.nlm.nih.gov/pmc/articles/PMC6182669/. Accessed 8 Jul. 2020.

[211] "Non-Celiac Gluten/Wheat Sensitivity | Celiac Disease ...." https://celiac.org/about-celiac-disease/related-conditions/non-celiac-wheat-gluten-sensitivity/. Accessed 8 Jul. 2020.

[212] "Wheat Belly: Lose the Wheat, Lose the Weight, and Find Your ...." https://www.amazon.com/Wheat-Belly-Lose-Weight-Health/dp/1609614798. Accessed 8 Jul. 2020.

[213] "Grain Brain: The Surprising Truth about Wheat ... - Amazon.com." https://www.amazon.com/Grain-Brain-Surprising-Sugar-Your-Killers/dp/031623480X. Accessed 8 Jul. 2020.

[214] "Testing for gluten-related disorders in clinical practice: The ...." https://www.ncbi.nlm.nih.gov/pmc/articles/PMC3088693/. Accessed 8 Jul. 2020.

[215] "Assessing of Celiac Disease and Nonceliac Gluten Sensitivity." 29 Apr. 2015, https://www.ncbi.nlm.nih.gov/pmc/articles/PMC4429206/. Accessed 8 Jul. 2020.

[216] "A structural basis for food allergy: the role of cross-reactivity.." https://www.ncbi.nlm.nih.gov/pubmed/18188023. Accessed 8 Jul. 2020.

[217] "Review Article: The Diagnosis and Management of Food ...."
14 Oct. 2014, https://pubmed.ncbi.nlm.nih.gov/25316115/.
Accessed 8 Jul. 2020.

[218] "Food Allergy: Separating the Science From the Mythology."
https://pubmed.ncbi.nlm.nih.gov/20606633. Accessed 8 Jul. 2020.

[219] "Oral Tolerance to Food Protein - PubMed." 8 Feb. 2012, https://
pubmed.ncbi.nlm.nih.gov/22318493. Accessed 8 Jul. 2020.

[220] "Detection of IgE, IgG, IgA and IgM antibodies against raw an."
12 May. 2009, https://pubmed.ncbi.nlm.nih.gov/19435515.
Accessed 8 Jul. 2020.

[221] "The Evolution of Food Immune Reactivity Testing - PubMed."
https://pubmed.ncbi.nlm.nih.gov/25599182/. Accessed 8 Jul. 2020.

[222] "Commercially available glutenases: a potential hazard in ...." 2
Apr. 2017, https://www.ncbi.nlm.nih.gov/pmc/articles/
PMC5424869/. Accessed 8 Jul. 2020.

[223] "A Food-Grade Enzyme Preparation With Modest Gluten ...." 21
Jul. 2009, https://pubmed.ncbi.nlm.nih.gov/19621078/. Accessed 8
Jul. 2020.

[224] "Neuromuscular diseases associated with antigliadin ... - NCBI."
https://www.ncbi.nlm.nih.gov/pubmed/15938571. Accessed 8 Jul.
2020.

[225] "Antigliadin antibodies in migraine patients. - NCBI." https://
www.ncbi.nlm.nih.gov/pubmed/9350395. Accessed 8 Jul. 2020.

[226] "Involvement of gut microbiota in the development of low-grade
...." https://www.ncbi.nlm.nih.gov/pmc/articles/PMC3463487/.
Accessed 10 Jul. 2020.

227 "Early Life Stress Alters Behavior, Immunity, and Microbiota in ...." 1 Feb. 2009, https://pubmed.ncbi.nlm.nih.gov/18723164/. Accessed 10 Jul. 2020.

228 "Antibiotic Exposure by 6 Months and Asthma and Allergy at 6 ...." 29 Dec. 2010, https://www.ncbi.nlm.nih.gov/pmc/articles/ PMC3105273/. Accessed 8 Jul. 2020.

229 "Thyroid receptors in the rat brain. - NCBI." https:// www.ncbi.nlm.nih.gov/pubmed/1502339. Accessed 8 Jul. 2020.

230 "Thyroid hormones: beneficial or deleterious for bone? - NCBI." https://www.ncbi.nlm.nih.gov/pubmed/14667131. Accessed 8 Jul. 2020.

231 "[Thyroid-intestinal Motility Interactions Summary] - PubMed." https://pubmed.ncbi.nlm.nih.gov/15788986/. Accessed 8 Jul. 2020.

232 "Glucoregulatory function of thyroid hormones: role of ... - NCBI." https://www.ncbi.nlm.nih.gov/pubmed/2563199. Accessed 8 Jul. 2020.

233 "Viruses and thyroiditis: an update - NCBI." 12 Jan. 2009, https://www.ncbi.nlm.nih.gov/pmc/articles/PMC2654877/. Accessed 8 Jul. 2020.

234 "The effects of thyroid hormones on the formation of stress ...." https://www.ncbi.nlm.nih.gov/pubmed/3945072. Accessed 8 Jul. 2020.

235 "Chemical Contamination and the Thyroid - PubMed." https:// pubmed.ncbi.nlm.nih.gov/25294013/. Accessed 8 Jul. 2020.

236 "Healing Spices: How to Use 50 Everyday and ... - Amazon.com." https://www.amazon.com/Healing-Spices-Everyday-Exotic-Disease/dp/1402776632. Accessed 8 Jul. 2020.

237 "Autoimmune Disease List • AARDA." https://www.aarda.org/diseaselist/. Accessed 8 Jul. 2020.

Chapter 8

238 "Effectiveness of Adjunctive Antidepressant Treatment for ...." 26 Apr. 2007, https://www.nejm.org/doi/pdf/10.1056/NEJMoa064135. Accessed 8 Jul. 2020.

239 "Stigma and the Toll of Addiction | NEJM." 2 Apr. 2020, https://www.nejm.org/doi/full/10.1056/NEJMp1917360. Accessed 8 Jul. 2020.

240 "Effectiveness of Adjunctive Antidepressant Treatment ... - Nejm." 26 Apr. 2007, https://www.nejm.org/doi/full/10.1056/nejmoa064135. Accessed 8 Jul. 2020.

241 "DNA Methylation and the Potential Role of Methyl-Containing ...." 16 Nov. 2017, https://www.ncbi.nlm.nih.gov/pmc/articles/PMC5733941/. Accessed 8 Jul. 2020.

242 "Methyl Donor Micronutrients that Modify DNA Methylation and ...." 13 Mar. 2019, https://www.ncbi.nlm.nih.gov/pmc/articles/PMC6471069/. Accessed 8 Jul. 2020.

243 "Meta-analysis of epigenome-wide association studies in ...." 23 Apr. 2019, https://www.nature.com/articles/s41467-019-09671-3. Accessed 8 Jul. 2020.

244 "Alzheimer's Disease Is Type 3 Diabetes–Evidence Reviewed." https://www.ncbi.nlm.nih.gov/pmc/articles/PMC2769828/. Accessed 8 Jul. 2020.

245 "Ubiquinol-10 Supplementation Activates Mitochondria ... - NCBI." https://www.ncbi.nlm.nih.gov/pmc/articles/PMC4025630/. Accessed 8 Jul. 2020.

246 "The Methylation, Neurotransmitter, and Antioxidant ... - PubMed." https://pubmed.ncbi.nlm.nih.gov/18950248/. Accessed 8 Jul. 2020.

247 "Environmental chemicals and DNA methylation in adults: a ...." 29 Apr. 2015, https://www.ncbi.nlm.nih.gov/pmc/articles/ PMC4433069/. Accessed 8 Jul. 2020.

248 "Understanding Epigenetic Effects of Endocrine Disrupting ...." https://pubmed.ncbi.nlm.nih.gov/28842957. Accessed 8 Jul. 2020.

249 "Effects of endocrine disrupting chemicals on in vitro global ...." https://www.sciencedirect.com/science/article/pii/ S0887233313000921. Accessed 8 Jul. 2020.

250 "DNA methylation disruption reshapes the hematopoietic ...." 23 Mar. 2020, https://www.nature.com/articles/s41588-020-0595-4. Accessed 8 Jul. 2020.

251 "DNA methylation is globally disrupted and ... - NCBI - NIH." https://www.ncbi.nlm.nih.gov/pubmed/24298892. Accessed 8 Jul. 2020.

252 "Methylcobalamin induces a long-lasting enhancement ... - NCBI." https://www.ncbi.nlm.nih.gov/pubmed/7675316. Accessed 10 Jul. 2020.

253 "Regulation of murine T-lymphocyte function by spleen cell ...." https://www.ncbi.nlm.nih.gov/pubmed/1294623. Accessed 10 Jul. 2020.

254 "Behavioral Effects of Dietary Neurotransmitter Precursors ...." https://pubmed.ncbi.nlm.nih.gov/8811719/. Accessed 10 Jul. 2020.

255 "Nonalcoholic fatty liver disease. - NCBI." https://www.ncbi.nlm.nih.gov/pubmed/16770927. Accessed 10 Jul. 2020.

256 "Behavioral Effects of Dietary Neurotransmitter Precursors ...." https://pubmed.ncbi.nlm.nih.gov/8811719/. Accessed 10 Jul. 2020.

257 "Association study of the nicotinic acetylcholine receptor α4 ...." 14 May. 2007, https://www.ncbi.nlm.nih.gov/pmc/articles/PMC4833496/. Accessed 10 Jul. 2020.

258 "The Human Genome Project." 7 Oct. 2019, https://www.genome.gov/human-genome-project. Accessed 8 Jul. 2020.

259 "Epigenetics - Latest research and news | Nature." https://www.nature.com/subjects/epigenetics. Accessed 8 Jul. 2020.

260 "Epigenetics: The Science of Change - NCBI." https://www.ncbi.nlm.nih.gov/pmc/articles/PMC1392256/. Accessed 8 Jul. 2020.

261 "The Impact of Nutrition and Environmental Epigenetics on ...." 1 Nov. 2018, https://www.ncbi.nlm.nih.gov/pmc/articles/PMC6275017/. Accessed 8 Jul. 2020.

262 "Food as exposure: Nutritional epigenetics and the new ... - NCBI." 7 Mar. 2011, https://www.ncbi.nlm.nih.gov/pmc/articles/PMC3500842/. Accessed 8 Jul. 2020.

263 "APOE gene - Genetics Home Reference - NIH." 23 Jun. 2020, https://ghr.nlm.nih.gov/gene/APOE. Accessed 8 Jul. 2020.

264 "What APOE Means for Your Health | Cognitive Vitality ...." 16 Nov. 2016, https://www.alzdiscovery.org/cognitive-vitality/blog/what-apoe-means-for-your-health. Accessed 8 Jul. 2020.

265 "Is MTHFR polymorphism a risk factor for Alzheimer's ... - NCBI." 13 Apr. 2005, https://www.ncbi.nlm.nih.gov/pubmed/15830056. Accessed 8 Jul. 2020.

266 "Folate and Folic Acid in Pregnancy - American Pregnancy ...." https://americanpregnancy.org/infertility/folate-vs-folic-acid/. Accessed 8 Jul. 2020.

267 "General Information About NTDs, Folic Acid, and Folate | CDC." https://www.cdc.gov/ncbddd/folicacid/faqs/faqs-general-info.html. Accessed 8 Jul. 2020.

268 "Multivitamin Supplementation During Pregnancy: Emphasis ...." https://www.ncbi.nlm.nih.gov/pmc/articles/PMC3250974/. Accessed 8 Jul. 2020.

Chapter 9

269 "How To Know If Your Air Is Unhealthy | American Lung ...." https://www.lung.org/clean-air/at-home/how-to-know-if-your-air-is-unhealthy. Accessed 10 Jul. 2020.

270 "• U.S. per capita consumption of soft drinks, 2018 | Statista." 1 Jul. 2020, https://www.statista.com/statistics/306836/us-per-capita-consumption-of-soft-drinks/. Accessed 8 Jul. 2020.

271 "Consumption of Sugar Drinks in the United States ... - CDC."
https://www.cdc.gov/nchs/products/databriefs/db71.htm. Accessed
8 Jul. 2020.

272 "Relationship of Soft Drink Consumption to Global
Overweight ...." https://www.ncbi.nlm.nih.gov/pmc/articles/
PMC3828681/. Accessed 8 Jul. 2020.

273 "Omega-3 Fatty Acids and Inflammatory Processes - NCBI." 18
Mar. 2010, https://www.ncbi.nlm.nih.gov/pmc/articles/
PMC3257651/. Accessed 8 Jul. 2020.

274 "Omega-6 Fatty Acids and Inflammation - PubMed." https://
pubmed.ncbi.nlm.nih.gov/29610056/. Accessed 8 Jul. 2020.

275 "Statins and All-Cause Mortality in High-Risk Primary
Prevention." 28 Jun. 2010, https://jamanetwork.com/journals/
jamainternalmedicine/fullarticle/416105. Accessed 8 Jul. 2020.

276 "Statin Use and Survival Outcomes in Elderly Patients With ...."
https://jamanetwork.com/journals/jamainternalmedicine/fullarticle/
486355. Accessed 8 Jul. 2020.

277 "Microwave ovens - World Health Organization." https://
www.who.int/peh-emf/publications/facts/info_microwaves/en/.
Accessed 8 Jul. 2020.

278 "Paleolithic Diets as a Model for Prevention and Treatment
of ...." https://pubmed.ncbi.nlm.nih.gov/22262579/. Accessed 10
Jul. 2020.

279 "Paleolithic Diet - StatPearls - NCBI Bookshelf." https://
www.ncbi.nlm.nih.gov/books/NBK482457/. Accessed 10 Jul. 2020.

[280] "Efficacy of the Autoimmune Protocol Diet for Inflammatory ...." 29 Aug. 2017, https://www.ncbi.nlm.nih.gov/pmc/articles/PMC5647120/. Accessed 10 Jul. 2020.

[281] "A Periodic Diet That Mimics Fasting Promotes Multi-System ...." 18 Jun. 2015, https://pubmed.ncbi.nlm.nih.gov/26094889/. Accessed 10 Jul. 2020.

[282] "Fasting-mimicking diet promotes Ngn3-driven β-cell ...." https://www.ncbi.nlm.nih.gov/pmc/articles/PMC5357144/. Accessed 10 Jul. 2020.

[283] "Effects of Intermittent Fasting on Health, Aging, and Disease ...." 26 Dec. 2019, https://www.nejm.org/doi/full/10.1056/nejmra1905136. Accessed 10 Jul. 2020.

Chapter 10

[284] "Repeated Sauna Therapy Attenuates Ventricular Remodeling ...." https://pubmed.ncbi.nlm.nih.gov/21622828/. Accessed 10 Jul. 2020.

[285] "Sauna Detoxification - Infrared Sauna Detox Benefits ...." 19 Nov. 2009, https://www.sunlighten.com/infrared-sauna-health-benefits/detoxification/. Accessed 10 Jul. 2020.

[286] "Clinical Effects of Regular Dry Sauna Bathing: A Systematic ...." 24 Apr. 2018, https://www.ncbi.nlm.nih.gov/pmc/articles/PMC5941775/. Accessed 10 Jul. 2020.

[287] "A study of thyroidal response to thyrotropin (TSH) in ...." https://www.ncbi.nlm.nih.gov/pubmed/2484874. Accessed 10 Jul. 2020.

288 "[The influence of treatment with substitutive or suppressive ...." https://www.researchgate.net/publication/ 7259178_The_influence_of_treatment_with_substitutive_or_suppre ssive_doses_of_thyroxine_on_biochemical_bone_turnover_markers . Accessed 10 Jul. 2020.

289 "Change of Bone Mineral Density and Biochemical Markers of ...." 31 Aug. 2015, https://www.ncbi.nlm.nih.gov/pmc/articles/ PMC4572035/. Accessed 10 Jul. 2020.

290 "Removal of Dental Amalgam Decreases anti-TPO and anti-Tg ...." https://pubmed.ncbi.nlm.nih.gov/16804512/. Accessed 10 Jul. 2020.

291 "Phenotypic Dichotomy Following Developmental Exposure to ...." 25 May. 2009, https://pubmed.ncbi.nlm.nih.gov/19433254/. Accessed 10 Jul. 2020.

292 "Risk of Brain Tumors From Wireless Phone Use - PubMed." https://pubmed.ncbi.nlm.nih.gov/21084892/. Accessed 10 Jul. 2020.

293 "Mobile Phone Use and Brain Tumours in the CERENAT Case ...." https://pubmed.ncbi.nlm.nih.gov/24816517/. Accessed 10 Jul. 2020.

294 "Cell phones and brain tumors: A review including the long term." https://pubmed.ncbi.nlm.nih.gov/19328536/. Accessed 10 Jul. 2020.

295 "Impact of Long-Term RF-EMF on Oxidative Stress and ...." 19 Jul. 2018, https://www.ncbi.nlm.nih.gov/pmc/articles/ PMC6073444/. Accessed 8 Jul. 2020.

[296] "Extremely low frequency electromagnetic field exposure and ...." 21 May. 2018, https://bmcneurosci.biomedcentral.com/articles/10.1186/s12868-018-0432-1. Accessed 8 Jul. 2020.

[297] "84,000 Chemicals on the Market, Only 1% Have Been Tested ...." 6 Jul. 2015, https://www.ecowatch.com/84-000-chemicals-on-the-market-only-1-have-been-tested-for-safety-1882062458.html. Accessed 8 Jul. 2020.

[298] "Bisphenol A and its analogs: Do their metabolites have ...." https://pubmed.ncbi.nlm.nih.gov/27771500/. Accessed 10 Jul. 2020.

[299] "Bisphenol A: An Endocrine Disruptor With Widespread ...." https://pubmed.ncbi.nlm.nih.gov/21605673/. Accessed 10 Jul. 2020.

[300] "The Toxic Effects of Xenobiotics on the Health of Humans and ...." 29 Mar. 2017, https://www.ncbi.nlm.nih.gov/pmc/articles/PMC5390638/. Accessed 8 Jul. 2020.

[301] "Chemical transformation of xenobiotics by the human gut ...." 23 Jun. 2017, https://science.sciencemag.org/content/356/6344/eaag2770.full. Accessed 8 Jul. 2020.

[302] "How Sleep Clears the Brain | National Institutes of Health (NIH)." 28 Oct. 2013, https://www.nih.gov/news-events/nih-research-matters/how-sleep-clears-brain. Accessed 8 Jul. 2020.

[303] "The Lymphatic System in Health and Disease - NCBI." https://www.ncbi.nlm.nih.gov/pmc/articles/PMC3572233/. Accessed 8 Jul. 2020.

[304] "The New Era of the Lymphatic System: No Longer Secondary ...." https://www.ncbi.nlm.nih.gov/pmc/articles/PMC3312397/. Accessed 8 Jul. 2020.

305 "Psychological Stress and Susceptibility to the Common Cold." 29 Aug. 1991, https://pubmed.ncbi.nlm.nih.gov/1713648/. Accessed 10 Jul. 2020.

306 "Irritable Bowel Syndrome, Anxiety, and Depression: What Are ...." https://pubmed.ncbi.nlm.nih.gov/12108820/. Accessed 10 Jul. 2020.

307 "Chronic Stress and Health Among Parents of Children With ...." https://pubmed.ncbi.nlm.nih.gov/20592593. Accessed 10 Jul. 2020.

308 "Cerebral Glucose Metabolism in Adults with Hyperactivity of ...." 15 Nov. 1990, https://www.nejm.org/doi/full/10.1056/nejm199011153232001. Accessed 10 Jul. 2020.

309 "Screening children with severe short stature for celiac disease ...." 19 Mar. 2010, https://www.ncbi.nlm.nih.gov/pubmed/20422329. Accessed 10 Jul. 2020.

Chapter 11

310 "Effect of magnitopuncture on sympathetic and ... - NCBI." 15 Nov. 2002, https://www.ncbi.nlm.nih.gov/pubmed/12527970. Accessed 10 Jul. 2020.

311 "Sympathetic Nerve Activity After Acupuncture in Humans." https://pubmed.ncbi.nlm.nih.gov/9539670/. Accessed 10 Jul. 2020.

312 "The effect of acupuncture on blood pressure: the interrelation ...." https://www.ncbi.nlm.nih.gov/pubmed/6135303. Accessed 10 Jul. 2020.

313 "Modulatory effect of acupuncture on the cardiovascular system ...." https://www.ncbi.nlm.nih.gov/pubmed/7902640. Accessed 10 Jul. 2020.

314 "Effect of Sensory Stimulation (Acupuncture) on Sympathetic ...." https://pubmed.ncbi.nlm.nih.gov/10683506/. Accessed 10 Jul. 2020.

315 "Acupuncture Induced Anaesthesia: Fiction Or Fact? - SAGE ...." https://journals.sagepub.com/doi/pdf/10.1136/ aim.11.2.55. Accessed 10 Jul. 2020.

316 "Perioperative acupuncture medicine: a novel concept instead ...." 20 Mar. 2019, https://www.ncbi.nlm.nih.gov/pmc/ articles/PMC6416101/. Accessed 10 Jul. 2020.

317 "Acupuncture--from Empiricism to Science: Functional ...." https://pubmed.ncbi.nlm.nih.gov/8569551. Accessed 10 Jul. 2020.

318 "Methods of evaluation of autonomic nervous system function." 9 Mar. 2010, https://www.ncbi.nlm.nih.gov/pmc/articles/ PMC3278937/. Accessed 10 Jul. 2020.

319 "Acupuncture: In Depth | NCCIH." https://www.nccih.nih.gov/ health/acupuncture-in-depth. Accessed 8 Jul. 2020.

320 "Bone changes due to pulses of direct electric microcurrent.." https://www.ncbi.nlm.nih.gov/pubmed/4628347. Accessed 10 Jul. 2020.

321 "Evaluation of microcurrent electrical nerve stimulation (MENS ...." https://www.ncbi.nlm.nih.gov/pubmed/19089032. Accessed 10 Jul. 2020.

322 "Effects of Microcurrent Treatment on Perceived Pain and ...." https://www.ncbi.nlm.nih.gov/pmc/articles/PMC1319813/. Accessed 10 Jul. 2020.

323 "Electro-membrane Microcurrent Therapy Reduces Signs and ...." https://pubmed.ncbi.nlm.nih.gov/11932567/. Accessed 10 Jul. 2020.

324 "Negative Pressure Wound Therapy Versus Microcurrent ...." https://pubmed.ncbi.nlm.nih.gov/30975055. Accessed 10 Jul. 2020.

325 "Microcurrent stimulation activates the circadian machinery in ...." 28 May. 2019, https://www.sciencedirect.com/science/article/pii/S0006291X19302037. Accessed 10 Jul. 2020.

326 "Microcurrent technology for rapid relief of sinus pain: a ... - NCBI." 22 Jan. 2019, https://www.ncbi.nlm.nih.gov/pmc/articles/PMC6590214/. Accessed 10 Jul. 2020.

327 "Martorell's Ulcer Successfully Treated by Wireless ... - NCBI." https://www.ncbi.nlm.nih.gov/pubmed/30653186. Accessed 10 Jul. 2020.

328 "Low-intensity microcurrent therapy promotes regeneration of ...." 12 Nov. 2018, https://www.ncbi.nlm.nih.gov/pubmed/30418167. Accessed 10 Jul. 2020.

329 "Microcurrent as an Adjunct Therapy to Accelerate Chronic ...." https://pubmed.ncbi.nlm.nih.gov/29738296/. Accessed 10 Jul. 2020.

330 "Therapeutic Effect of Microcurrent on Calf Muscle Atrophy in ...." https://pubmed.ncbi.nlm.nih.gov/29466826/. Accessed 10 Jul. 2020.

331 "Effects of Integrated Treatment With LED and Microcurrent on ...." 12 Jun. 2018, https://pubmed.ncbi.nlm.nih.gov/29950771/. Accessed 10 Jul. 2020.

332 "Effects of microcurrent and cryotherapy on C-reactive protein ...." 27 Jan. 2018, https://www.ncbi.nlm.nih.gov/pubmed/29410562. Accessed 10 Jul. 2020.

333 "Bioelectrical signals improve cardiac function and modify gene." 30 Jun. 2017, https://www.ncbi.nlm.nih.gov/pubmed/28772035. Accessed 10 Jul. 2020.

334 "Short-term microcurrent electrical neuromuscular stimulation ...." https://www.ncbi.nlm.nih.gov/pubmed/28658177. Accessed 10 Jul. 2020.

335 "Microcurrent stimulation promotes reverse remodelling in ...." 6 Jan. 2016, https://www.ncbi.nlm.nih.gov/pmc/articles/PMC5064659/. Accessed 10 Jul. 2020.

336 "Efficacy of Pulsed Low-Intensity Electric Neuromuscular ...." https://pubmed.ncbi.nlm.nih.gov/27358158. Accessed 10 Jul. 2020.

337 "Microcurrent stimulation promotes reverse remodelling in ...." 6 Jan. 2016, https://www.ncbi.nlm.nih.gov/pmc/articles/PMC5064659/. Accessed 10 Jul. 2020.

338 "Efficacy of Pulsed Low-Intensity Electric Neuromuscular ...." https://pubmed.ncbi.nlm.nih.gov/27358158. Accessed 10 Jul. 2020.

339 "Effects of microcurrent therapy on excisional elastic cartilage ...." https://www.ncbi.nlm.nih.gov/pubmed/27138327. Accessed 10 Jul. 2020.

340 "Enhancement of delay eyelid conditioning by microcurrent ...." 13 Jan. 2016, https://www.ncbi.nlm.nih.gov/pubmed/26998030. Accessed 10 Jul. 2020.

341 "[The Influence of Electrical Stimulation on the Peripheral ...." https://pubmed.ncbi.nlm.nih.gov/26595968. Accessed 10 Jul. 2020.

342 "Microcurrent Electrical Neuromuscular Stimulation Facilitates ...." 8 May. 2015, https://www.ncbi.nlm.nih.gov/pmc/articles/PMC4424458/. Accessed 10 Jul. 2020.

343 "Effects of low-frequency electrical stimulation on cumulative ...." 9 Jan. 2015, https://www.ncbi.nlm.nih.gov/pmc/articles/PMC4305535/. Accessed 10 Jul. 2020.

344 "Efficacy of microcurrent therapy in infants with congenital ...." 15 Nov. 2013, https://www.researchgate.net/publication/258635481_Efficacy_of_microcurrent_therapy_in_infants_with_congenital_muscular_torticollis_involving_the_entire_sternocleidomastoid_muscle_A_randomized_placebo-controlled_trial. Accessed 10 Jul. 2020.

345 "Effect of Biphasic Electrical Current Stimulation on IL-1β ...." 15 Oct. 2013, https://pubmed.ncbi.nlm.nih.gov/23823576/. Accessed 10 Jul. 2020.

346 "The Use of Targeted MicroCurrent Therapy in Postoperative ...." https://pubmed.ncbi.nlm.nih.gov/23446501/. Accessed 10 Jul. 2020.

347 "Use of wireless microcurrent stimulation for the treatment of ...." https://www.ncbi.nlm.nih.gov/pubmed/23263389. Accessed 10 Jul. 2020.

348 "[The role of microcurrent reflexotherapy in combination ... - NCBI." https://www.ncbi.nlm.nih.gov/pubmed/23210360. Accessed 10 Jul. 2020.

349 "Microcurrent Therapy in the Management of Chronic Tennis ...." https://pubmed.ncbi.nlm.nih.gov/22147671/. Accessed 10 Jul. 2020.

350 "Microcurrent Transcutaneous Electric Nerve Stimulation in ...." https://pubmed.ncbi.nlm.nih.gov/21627767/. Accessed 10 Jul. 2020.

351 "[The Influence of Electrical Stimulation on the Peripheral ...." https://pubmed.ncbi.nlm.nih.gov/26595968. Accessed 10 Jul. 2020.

352 "The Use of Targeted MicroCurrent Therapy in Postoperative ...." https://pubmed.ncbi.nlm.nih.gov/23446501/. Accessed 10 Jul. 2020.

353 "Use of wireless microcurrent stimulation for the treatment of ...." https://www.ncbi.nlm.nih.gov/pubmed/23263389. Accessed 10 Jul. 2020.

354 "[The role of microcurrent reflexotherapy in combination ... - NCBI." https://www.ncbi.nlm.nih.gov/pubmed/23210360. Accessed 10 Jul. 2020.

355 "Microcurrent Therapy in the Management of Chronic Tennis ...." https://pubmed.ncbi.nlm.nih.gov/22147671/. Accessed 10 Jul. 2020.

356 "Microcurrent Transcutaneous Electric Nerve Stimulation in ...." https://pubmed.ncbi.nlm.nih.gov/21627767/. Accessed 10 Jul. 2020.

357 "The efficacy of frequency specific microcurrent therapy on ...." https://bjsm.bmj.com/content/45/2/e3.1. Accessed 10 Jul. 2020.

358 "Effectiveness of Microcurrent Therapy as a Constituent of Post ...." 8 Jun. 2010, https://pubmed.ncbi.nlm.nih.gov/20533147/. Accessed 10 Jul. 2020.

359 "Effectiveness of transcutaneous electrical nerve stimulation ...." https://www.ncbi.nlm.nih.gov/pubmed/20427917. Accessed 10 Jul. 2020.

360 "The efficacy of frequency specific microcurrent therapy on ...." https://bjsm.bmj.com/content/45/2/e3.1. Accessed 10 Jul. 2020.

361 "Visceral and Somatic Disorders: Tissue Softening with ... - NCBI." https://www.ncbi.nlm.nih.gov/pmc/articles/PMC3576917/. Accessed 10 Jul. 2020.

362 "Effects of low-frequency electrical stimulation on cumulative ...." 9 Jan. 2015, https://www.ncbi.nlm.nih.gov/pmc/articles/PMC4305535/. Accessed 10 Jul. 2020.

363 "Frequency-Specific Microcurrent for Treatment of ... - PubMed." https://pubmed.ncbi.nlm.nih.gov/30664049/. Accessed 10 Jul. 2020.

Chapter 12

364 "Cervical Spine Manipulation Alters Sensorimotor Integration ...." https://pubmed.ncbi.nlm.nih.gov/17137836/. Accessed 10 Jul. 2020.

365 "Neck Muscle Afferents Influence Oromotor and ... - PubMed." https://pubmed.ncbi.nlm.nih.gov/24595534/. Accessed 10 Jul. 2020.

366 "A hypothesis of chronic back pain: ligament subfailure injuries ...." 27 Jul. 2005, https://www.ncbi.nlm.nih.gov/pmc/articles/PMC3489327/. Accessed 10 Jul. 2020.

367 "Mechanoreceptors in Diseased Cervical Intervertebral Disc ...." 15 Apr. 2017, https://pubmed.ncbi.nlm.nih.gov/27438387. Accessed 10 Jul. 2020.

368 "Measureable Changes in the Neuro-Endocrinal Mechanism ...." https://pubmed.ncbi.nlm.nih.gov/26464145/. Accessed 10 Jul. 2020.

369 "An immunohistochemical study of mechanoreceptors ... - NCBI." 26 Mar. 2020, https://www.ncbi.nlm.nih.gov/pubmed/20347312. Accessed 10 Jul. 2020.

370 "Cerebral Metabolic Changes in Men After Chiropractic Spinal ...." https://pubmed.ncbi.nlm.nih.gov/22314714/. Accessed 10 Jul. 2020.

371 "Manipulation of Dysfunctional Spinal Joints Affects ... - PubMed." https://pubmed.ncbi.nlm.nih.gov/27047694. Accessed 10 Jul. 2020.

372 "The Vagus Nerve Can Predict and Possibly Modulate Non ...." 19 Oct. 2018, https://www.ncbi.nlm.nih.gov/pmc/articles/PMC6210465/. Accessed 10 Jul. 2020.

373 "In Vivo Effects of Low Level Laser Therapy on ... - PubMed." https://pubmed.ncbi.nlm.nih.gov/19291752/. Accessed 10 Jul. 2020.

374 "Laser biostimulation of wound healing: bioimpedance ... - NCBI." https://www.ncbi.nlm.nih.gov/pubmed/27371448. Accessed 10 Jul. 2020.

375 "Low intensity 635 nm diode laser irradiation inhibits fibroblast ...." 10 Dec. 2015, https://www.ncbi.nlm.nih.gov/pubmed/26660509. Accessed 10 Jul. 2020.

376 "Low-Level Laser Therapy at 635 Nm for Treatment of Chronic ...." 10 Mar. 2015, https://pubmed.ncbi.nlm.nih.gov/25769363. Accessed 10 Jul. 2020.

377 "Body Contouring Using 635-nm Low Level Laser Therapy." https://pubmed.ncbi.nlm.nih.gov/24049928. Accessed 10 Jul. 2020.

378 "Low-level Laser Therapy and Vibration Therapy for ... - PubMed." https://pubmed.ncbi.nlm.nih.gov/23888254. Accessed 10 Jul. 2020.

379 "Low-level laser irradiation alters cardiac cytokine expression ...." 24 Feb. 2011, https://www.ncbi.nlm.nih.gov/pubmed/21348574. Accessed 10 Jul. 2020.

380 "Effects of photobiomodulation therapy in aerobic endurance ...." https://www.ncbi.nlm.nih.gov/pubmed/31045769. Accessed 10 Jul. 2020.

381 "Laserpuncture Increases Serum Concentration of Insulin-Like ...." 17 Dec. 2018, https://www.ncbi.nlm.nih.gov/pmc/articles/PMC6338566/. Accessed 10 Jul. 2020.

382 "Efficiency of hyperuricemia correction by low level laser ...." https://www.ncbi.nlm.nih.gov/pubmed/30448802. Accessed 10 Jul. 2020.

383 "Is Low-Level Laser Therapy Effective in Acute or Chronic Low ...." https://pubmed.ncbi.nlm.nih.gov/20414695/. Accessed 10 Jul. 2020.

384 "Transmeatal Cochlear Laser (TCL) Treatment of ... - PubMed." https://pubmed.ncbi.nlm.nih.gov/14505199/. Accessed 10 Jul. 2020.

385 "Effects of Low-Level Laser Therapy on Malignant Cells: In ...." https://pubmed.ncbi.nlm.nih.gov/11902350/. Accessed 10 Jul. 2020.

386 "Effects on the mitosis of normal and tumor cells induced by ...." https://pubmed.ncbi.nlm.nih.gov/10495304/. Accessed 10 Jul. 2020.

387 "The impact of wavelengths of LED light-therapy on endothelial ...." 6 Sep. 2017, https://www.nature.com/articles/ s41598-017-11061-y. Accessed 10 Jul. 2020.

388 "A Double-Blind, Placebo-Controlled Randomized Evaluation ...." https://pubmed.ncbi.nlm.nih.gov/28682676/. Accessed 10 Jul. 2020.

389 "Mesenchymal Stem Cells Synergize with 635, 532, and 405 ...." https://www.ncbi.nlm.nih.gov/pubmed/27244220. Accessed 10 Jul. 2020.

390 "Influence of low-level laser (LLL) on ...." https:// www.ncbi.nlm.nih.gov/pubmed/31053447. Accessed 10 Jul. 2020.

391 "Effects of photobiomodulation therapy in aerobic endurance ." https://www.ncbi.nlm.nih.gov/pubmed/31045769. Accessed 10 Jul. 2020.

392 "Wound-healing effects of 635-nm low-level laser therapy on ...." https://www.ncbi.nlm.nih.gov/pubmed/30244401. Accessed 10 Jul. 2020.

393 "Effect of photobiomodulation on neural differentiation ... - NCBI." 19 Sep. 2018, https://www.ncbi.nlm.nih.gov/pubmed/ 30232645. Accessed 10 Jul. 2020.

394 "Red (635 Nm), Near-Infrared (808 Nm) and Violet-Blue (405 ...." 3 Jul. 2018, https://pubmed.ncbi.nlm.nih.gov/29970828/. Accessed 10 Jul. 2020.

395 "Effectiveness of Low Level Laser Therapy for Treating Male ...." https://pubmed.ncbi.nlm.nih.gov/29806585/. Accessed 10 Jul. 2020.